Happy Birthday
Steve
Love Mom & Dad.
1989 -

Dr. Andy

Answers Your Everyday Medical Questions

Dr. Andy

Answers Your Everyday Medical Questions

Andrew P. Morley, Jr., M.D.

OLIVER NELSON

A DIVISION OF THOMAS NELSON PUBLISHERS
Nashville • Atlanta • Camden • New York

Copyright © 1986 by Andrew P. Morley, Jr.

All rights reserved. Written permission must be secured from the publisher to use or reproduce any part of this book, except for brief quotations in critical reviews or articles.

Published in Nashville, Tennessee, by Oliver-Nelson Books, a division of Thomas Nelson, Inc., Publishers, and distributed in Canada by Lawson Falle, Ltd., Cambridge, Ontario.

Printed in the United States of America.

Library of Congress Cataloging-in-Publication Data

Morley, Andrew P.
  Dr. Andy answers your everyday medical questions.

  Includes index.
  1. Medicine, Popular—Miscellanea. I. Title.
RC81.M875 1986   616   86-16337
ISBN 0-8407-9070-8

DEDICATION

To my loving wife, Debbie,
without whose understanding and patience
during my years of being a Media Doc
this book would not have been possible.

CONTENTS

INTRODUCTION

Your health is your responsibility. Happiness and a long and productive life are directly related to the choices you make about taking care of your health, and so it is important to learn as much as you can about how to achieve the best health possible.

Many of today's major health problems can be prevented. The chances of succumbing to one of our three greatest killers can be significantly reduced if only we would exercise regularly, eat sensibly, and stop smoking. Heart attacks, strokes, and many forms of cancer are largely preventable. The more you know about prevention, the better your chances will be.

One of the most common complaints I hear from my patients and from my listening audiences is that there are many questions they would like to ask their doctors but they never seem to have the opportunity. In *Dr. Andy Answers Your Everyday Medical Questions* I have tried to provide you with the basic information you need to begin your quest for a healthier life.

As you read, keep in mind that my answers to these questions are not intended to diagnosis your problems or to replace the relationship you have with your personal physician. No one could, or should, try to diagnose in a book. The information in this book is intended to help you understand health care, help you prevent certain diseases, and help you be better informed about taking care of yourself and your family when illness occurs.

Use the information in this book wisely, and always consult your personal physician when you have questions specific to your health.

1.

Blueprint for Good Health

INTRODUCTION

We all want to live long and happy lives. We also realize that achieving this goal is not easy. Numerous studies show us that the cornerstone for success in living long, happy, and productive lives is good health. But most of us take good health for granted and forget that good health is like anything else in life: we have to work for it. Nutrition, exercise, and good health habits are the keys to good health and good life.

Keeping our bodies healthy is somewhat like providing good maintenance for our cars. Cars need certain nutrients such as gas, oil, and water to function properly. The spark plugs need to be clean and synchronized. A well-tuned automobile satisfies our transportation needs with maximum efficiency.

Our bodies have similar needs. They need certain nutrients and maintenance to be "fine-tuned." And only when we are fine-tuned do we function at maximum capacity for long periods of time. So it is important that we all understand the influence that nutrition, exercise, and good personal health habits have on our present and future health.

NUTRITION

Why is good nutrition important?

Proper nutrition is vital for a long and healthy life. The foods you eat provide energy to carry on your daily activities and give the proper nutrients that maintain and repair your body tissues and help you fight off disease. *You are what you eat*. If your diet contains the proper

17

amounts of nutrients, your body will function properly and resist disease more efficiently. On the other hand, if your diet lacks certain essential nutrients or energy foods, your body certainly will not function properly and, like a poorly maintained car, will begin to break down faster.

What is a well-balanced diet?

A well-balanced diet includes the proper amounts of foods from the 4 basic food groups: (1) milk and milk products; (2) meat, fish, and poultry; (3) breads and cereals; and (4) fruits and vegetables. Each of these groups supplies something special to make your body function properly.

A review of most people's dietary habits reveals that they tend to lean more to 1 group than another; it is really unusual to find someone who has mastered the art of the well-balanced diet.

Of course, when you talk about your particular nutritional status, you must consider your age, body build, and any special health problems. But what is essential is that you understand how the 4 basic food groups relate to and work in a well-balanced diet and how changes in health and age can relate to changes in the balancing of these food groups.

THE 4 BASIC FOOD GROUPS

1. Milk and milk products

In addition to whole, skim, and low-fat milk, this group contains buttermilk, cheese, cottage cheese, yogurt, and ice cream. These foods provide calcium to build strong bones and teeth, protein to preserve and repair body tissue, and vitamin B-2 (riboflavin) to help maintain healthy skin.

This group is especially important at 2 different ages. As children grow, they need adequate amounts of calcium to maintain good strong bones and teeth. In underdeveloped countries, a major problem is that most children do not get the milk group nutrients. Recent advances in medicine and health have also taught us that it is critical for the elderly population to get adequate amounts from the milk group. Without an adequate supply of calcium, a wasting-away of bone tissue (osteoporosis) can occur.

How much food should you eat from the milk group? You should have at least 2 cups of milk, or the equivalent, each day; 1 cup milk provides about the same amount of calcium as 1 cup yogurt, 2 cups cottage cheese, and 1½ ounces regular cheese, or 1¾ cups ice cream. As long as you maintain amounts at this level, you are receiving a well-balanced diet from the milk group.

2. Meat, fish, and poultry

The meat group also includes representatives from the fish, chicken, and egg group. Eating 2 servings daily of poultry, lean meat, fish, eggs, peanut butter, nuts, soy extenders, dry beans, peas, or lentils provides the proper amount of nutrients from this group.

These foods provide protein for preserving and repairing body tissues, and iron and B vitamins for keeping the nervous system and skin healthy.

Individual servings that would provide the necessary requirements from the meat group include any of the following: 2 or 3 ounces cooked poultry, meat, or fish; 2 eggs; 4 teaspoons peanut butter, or ⅓ cup nuts.

There are certain advantages and disadvantages to utilizing certain representatives of this food group. The American Heart Association, for instance, recommends that people eat no more than 3 eggs per week because of the very high cholesterol content and its relationship to the development of heart disease. There has also been much discussion by the American Cancer Society regarding the proper diet in preventing cancer. Red meats seem to be related to potential increases in the incidence of cancer, and we should be cautious in increasing our consumption of red meats. We should also note that red meats are much higher in calories than the representatives from the fish and poultry groups. Red meat would supply adequate nutrients from the meat group, but if you are trying to lose weight, try to supply them from the fish and poultry area, instead.

3. Breads and cereals

This group provides carbohydrates for energy and the iron, B vitamins, and fiber necessary for digestion and elimination. We need at least 4 daily servings of representatives from the bread group, which includes bread, cereal, saltines, muffins, macaroni, noodles, spaghetti, and rice. There are advantages and disadvantages to particular representatives of the bread/cereal group. Whole-grain products have the greatest amounts of nutrients and fiber. The American Cancer Society tells us that an increase in the amount of fiber in our diet can significantly decrease our chances of developing cancer of the lower digestive tract. Bread made with white flour loses the fiber content during processing and is not as healthful as whole-grain breads and cereals.

Individual servings of this group that would satisfy daily requirements include 1 slice of bread, ¾ cup dry cereal, ½ cup cooked cereal, 5 saltines, 1 muffin, or ½ cup macaroni, noodles, rice, or spaghetti.

4. Fruits and vegetables

Fruits and vegetables are the primary providers of vitamin C, which is essential for maintaining healthy gums and skin, for healing wounds, for resisting infection, and for preventing bruises. Citrus fruits, melons, strawberries, apples, tomatoes, or potatoes are all rich in vitamin C. Juice, especially orange juice, is a good source of vitamin C, but it does not provide as much fiber as raw or cooked fruits and vegetables.

Green and deep yellow fruits and vegetables provide the vitamin A necessary for healthy eyes, skin, and hair and for resistance to infection. Representatives of this group include broccoli, spinach, turnip greens, pumpkin, carrots, and cantaloupe.

Because of the importance of vitamin A, vitamin C, and roughage, you should have at least 2 or more servings of fruits and vegetables each day from the vitamin C *and* vitamin A groups. Eating 4 servings of fruits and vegetables is a good daily guide (1 serving is ½ cup fruit, vegetable, or juice). A secret of good nutrition is obtaining the nutrients and energy needed from a wide variety of foods.

Do we have any special needs that are not met by the 4 basic food groups?

The 4 basic food groups provide the vast majority of the energy and nutrients our bodies need. However, some other special needs must be considered. Water, for example, does not have real food value, but it is an essential element of our diet. The body needs at least 4 8-ounce glasses of water per day to function properly. Some people say that they drink a lot of coffee or tea or perhaps even alcoholic beverages to satisfy their water needs. But few people realize that these substances are actually diuretics—they make the body *lose* water. So if you drink coffee, tea, or alcohol, your body really needs *more* than 4 glasses of water each day.

IDEAL BODY WEIGHT

What does my ideal body weight mean?

"Ideal body weight" simply refers to how much you should weigh, taking into consideration your age, sex, and body build. Studies show that people who keep their weight within that ideal range are much less prone to developing high blood pressure, heart disease, and diabetes. So it is critical not only to eat a properly balanced diet but also to tailor that diet so you either maintain or achieve an ideal body weight.

But can I calculate my ideal weight?

Doctors hear this question over and over again from many people, and there are 2 ways to find out exactly how much you should weigh. You can use a standard growth chart for adults, which establishes an average range according to sex, height, and body build. These charts can be obtained from your physician, public health department, or local nutritional experts, such as the Diabetes Foundation or the American Heart Association in your community.

But there's a simpler way, using a simple formula that anyone can calculate. The standard tells us that a 5′ woman should weigh approximately 100 pounds. For every inch above 5′, we add 4 pounds to get the ideal body weight of the woman, so a 5′6″ woman should weigh 124 pounds. For every inch below 5′, we subtract 4 pounds, making 84 pounds the ideal weight for a woman who is 4′8″. Note that these calculations apply to adults. The growth charts for children and young adults are more refined in detail and should be obtained from your physician.

Determining a man's ideal body weight is basically the same. However, in calculating a man's ideal body weight, use 5 pounds instead of 4. A man who is 5′ tall should weigh approximately 110 pounds. Therefore, a man who is 6′ tall should weigh approximately 170 pounds. Remember that body weights will fluctuate depending upon the bone size of the person.

How do I measure my bone size?

To determine if you are a large- or small-boned person, simply check your wrist. If you can place your thumb and index finger all the way around your wrist, your bones are probably of average size. If your fingers overlap, then you are probably a small-boned person. If your fingers do not touch (assuming there is no arthritis or deformity), you are probably a large-boned person. Once you have determined your bone size, then go back to your ideal body weight. If you are small-boned, subtract 5 pounds from your ideal body weight. If you are of average bone size, do not adjust the ideal figure. If you are large-boned, add 5 pounds to your calculated ideal weight.

Do ideal body weight and nutritional requirements change with age?

They certainly do. There are 2 main age groups that have special nutritional needs and different ideal body weights.

The 1st group includes adolescents. The eating patterns of adolescents have long been of major concern to parents and health professionals, since this is a time of intensive growth and hormonal changes. Because of the growth spurt and hormonal changes that take place, adolescents must get an adequate amount of protein and calcium needed for growth. Larger quantities of many vitamins are also needed to maintain the adequate body energy needed. Adolescence is also a time when good eating and dietary habits become a pattern that, if established correctly, can be carried on into later years. Unfortunately, adolescents have particular problems maintaining good nutrition because of very busy schedules and numerous activities. Often these factors contribute to or cause irregular eating habits. Food choices then become even more critical in this age group. Young female adolescents who have begun their menstrual cycles also need additional iron. And don't forget that young males need adequate amounts of iron because of the increase in lean body mass, or muscular structure.

Adolescents involved in sports will, of course, need more energy (calories) while adolescents whose interests are more sedentary will require less energy. Adolescents do not need special nutrient supplements. Parents of "underweight" adolescents constantly ask physicians how they can get the child's weight up to "normal." Unless this is a physical problem that makes the child feel bad, my general suggestion is to leave the child alone. A child who is relatively thin for his or her age at 14 could hit a growth spurt between 14 and 15 and end up overweight in a year or so. The best advice is not to be concerned with the adolescent's weight unless your physician advises you that the child is grossly over or under weight. It's more important to make sure a well-balanced diet is eaten.

The 4 basic food groups will provide a balanced diet for the adolescent: (1) meat and meat alternatives such as fish and poultry—2 servings a day; (2) fruits and vegetables, particularly those in the vitamin A and vitamin C groups—4 servings a day; (3) breads and cereals—4 servings a day; and (4) milk and milk products—3–4 cups a day of milk or 2–3 ounces of milk products.

Older people are in the 2nd age group that must consider special nutritional requirements. Older citizens must pay careful attention to diet because the aging process reduces the lean body mass or muscle mass, which increases the fat mass. In addition, most older Americans have a fairly sedate lifestyle, and with less exercise, they cannot burn off the calories they take in. Older people, therefore, require fewer calories each day.

Protein requirements do not appear to increase or decrease markedly with age. Calcium requirements, however, must be maintained or even increased.

Osteoporosis, a serious problem in older women, may be due in part to a chronic calcium deficiency. Requirements for elderly people may be such that even if the daily milk or milk product intake is approximately 2 glasses per day, calcium supplements may be necessary to prevent osteoporosis. We need to note here that vitamin D is essential for calcium taken in through diet or supplements to be transferred to the bones to increase bone strength. Studies show that elderly people have a lower level of circulating vitamin D. So, when supplements are given to an elderly person, vitamin D should be included.

Important also to this group is proper bowel function. Many older Americans complain of constipation, which could be related to lack of fiber or whole-grain in the diet. Older people need to increase the amount of fiber they take in, from whole-grain breads or cereals as well as raw fruits and vegetables. If this is not enough, fiber supplement products can be purchased across the counter. Adequate amounts of water also promote regular bowel function.

WEIGHT REDUCTION

What is the best way to lose weight?

The local corner bookstore and drugstore offer a large number of "remedies" for losing weight. However, anyone desiring to reach ideal body weight through dieting needs to understand a basic principle: the best diet decreases the amount of calories taken in and increases the amount of calories burned off. This seems like a very simple formula for losing weight—it is, in fact. It is also tried and true and results not only in reducing weight but in keeping that weight off.

I do not like the word *diet* because it implies something that you start and something that you eventually stop. Most people who are trying to lose weight need to realize that they don't need to diet; they need to change their eating habits. So we're talking about something that is permanent, not temporary. How do you change your eating habits? Well, do you know people who have gone on a diet and lost 15 or 20 pounds? Then they felt so good about their accomplishment that they went off the diet, and the pounds gradually came back. Why? Because even though their eating changed (temporarily), their eating habits did not. The habits that you pick up during your diet should be continued throughout the rest of your life. If you do this, your weight problem will

23

be permanently, not temporarily, cured. To maintain your normal body weight where it should be, a certain amount of calories are required each day. Your body needs these calories to promote energy for your daily activities and to maintain the proper growth that goes on no matter how old you are. The cells in the body are constantly being destroyed and are constantly being replaced by new cells.

But there are some basic outlines regarding the number of calories you should take in if you are trying to lose weight. In general, a daily intake of 1500 calories for men and 1000 calories for women induces satisfactory weight loss over an extended period of time. The key is to make sure that the calories are properly balanced among the 4 basic food groups. Maintaining this caloric intake should provide you with a fairly steady weight loss of approximately 1 to 2 pounds per week.

Can I use over-the-counter diet pills if I am trying to lose weight?

When we consider that obesity is a major American health problem, it's no wonder that we turn to almost anything to find the answer to the "battle of the bulge." People are looking for the quickest, most convenient way to lose weight—so they turn to diet pills. Most favor the over-the-counter pills that do not require a doctor's prescription. Over $20 million a year are spent on these chemicals.

The major component in these over-the-counter diet pills is phenylpropanolamine. Now that's a 50¢ word, but if it sounds rather familiar, that's because it is a stimulant similar to the amphetamines and also a major component in cold medications. Although it seems to decrease the appetite, it stimulates the heart and vascular system. If the recommended dose is exceeded, these pills can cause nervousness, anorexia, headache, increased heart rate, and elevated blood pressure.

These diet pills are considered safe when taken in doses of no more than 105 mg of phenylpropanolamine. However, I have strong questions about whether or not someone can lose weight and keep it off through the use of these aids. The overall effectiveness and safety of these medications are questionable.

If you choose over-the-counter diet pills, and I hope you don't, be sure to ask your physician or pharmacist about *any* unusual symptoms you might be experiencing. Also ask if you can take them with medication you might already be taking.

Are "fad diets" successful?

Millions of Americans spend millions of dollars annually just buying the books that explain many of the fad diets out today. Your neighborhood bookstore has shelf upon shelf of books proclaiming 1 diet or another to be the best. If you look up the word *fad* in *Webster's New Collegiate Dictionary,* you'll find the following definition: "a practice or interest followed for a time with exaggerated zeal; a craze." I think this definition sums up the effectiveness of fad diets. Everyone is looking for the quick fix. Regardless of what the advertisements tell you, there is no such thing as a miracle diet. Indeed, if there was, most people would not be changing to a different fad every year or so. I go back to the basic premise of losing weight: cut down the number of calories you take in and increase the number of calories you burn off through exercise. Remember that *diet* is a bad word. Dieting means something you start and something you'll stop. Add the word *fad* to that and not only are you starting something you eventually intend to stop, but you are starting something overzealously that, in the long run, will have little success.

We all know that certain types of diets, if followed correctly, are not dangerous to health. Many of us have lost weight on 1 diet or another. The major benefit of a particular diet is that you may be comfortable with it. Just like exercise, if you are not comfortable with the diet you're on, and are not enthusiastic about following it, you're not going to follow it and you're not going to lose weight.

The best way is to check with your physician to see if a particular diet program, whether or not it is a fad, is safe for you. If you do go on a fad diet and begin to feel bad or lose weight too rapidly, check with your physician immediately.

In the past, we have seen fad diets come and go. Some fad diets, such as the liquid protein diet of the mid-1970s, were reported in the press to be implicated in some deaths. Other diets are not quite this dramatic but should be examined with caution. Remember the statement: you are what you eat. If you are putting some crazy concoction into your body, your body is going to respond—perhaps violently.

What is some good advice on how to diet?

Don't expect dramatic and immediate results. It took a long time to get to the weight you are, and it will take a long time to get back to the weight you want or need to be. Some people's bodies have a greater tendency to gain and retain weight. If you are such a person, it is quite possible to lose that weight, but it takes a long time. If you are more than 30 pounds overweight, you probably should count on 6 months to a year to have that weight back to where you want it and be able to maintain it there.

A thorough review of the reasons people become overweight shows that many people use food as a substitute for displaced anger or stress;

they have learned to turn to the pleasure of eating to relieve tension and boredom. When you have an urge to snack to get an emotional lift, do something else. Remove yourself from the presence of food. Get outside, take a stroll, get some exercise, and do anything you need to do to break the association between stress and eating. Likewise, if you use eating as a substitute for depression, consult your physician on ways to relieve the depression.

Have a positive outlook. People who are successful over the long haul tell me that they get maximum success when they involve family and friends in their plan. If you are trying to lose weight, ask your family to support you and help you maintain a positive outlook. There will be times when your weight will reach a plateau and not change for a week or more, and that will be a very discouraging time for you. The positive support that family and friends can give you will help you over the hump to the next gradual drop in your weight.

Remember that some form of exercise is almost mandatory to lose weight. Regardless of the diet you use, combine it with some form of daily exercise such as jogging, aerobics, daily walks, or swimming. Learn the caloric content of common foods and restrict your intake to approximately 1000 to 1500 calories a day. Increasing exercise burns calories and excess stored fat.

How can I determine how much body fat I have?

To estimate your percentage of body fat, use the old thumb-and-forefinger pinch. Take your thumb and forefinger, and gently pinch your side just above the top of the hip. For men, if you pinched less than ½", score 10; ½" to ¾", score 5; ¾" to 1", score 3; more than 1", score 1. For women, if you pinched less than 1", score 10; 1" to 1½", score 5; 1½" to 2", score 3; more than 2", score 1.

If you scored 3 on this test, then your percentage of body fat is significant. In fact, if you scored 1 to 3 points, you may need to significantly improve your muscle tone before attempting any vigorous exercise program.

How many calories does it take to lose a pound?

It's been estimated that if you reduce your required calorie intake by 3500 calories, you will lose a pound. That means if you can manipulate your current food consumption over the span of a week and reduce your intake by 3500 calories (500 calories each day), you will lose approximately 1 pound. Reducing your diet by 500 calories a day may sound like a big chore, but it is surprisingly simple. For example, if you are accustomed to eating 10 slices of bread a week, simply reducing that to

5 slices will cut your caloric intake from bread alone in half. If you eat dessert with each evening meal, try eating dessert with only 3 meals per week. Again, this will cut your weekly caloric intake from desserts almost in half. A lot of people lose a significant amount of weight simply by following this basic principle. They do not significantly change the types of food they eat, but they decrease the amounts.

VITAMINS AND MINERALS

If I'm on a diet, do I need to take vitamins?

If your caloric intake is less than 1500 calories per day, you probably need to supplement your diet. Check with your physician for an appropriate vitamin/mineral preparation.

Why are vitamins and minerals necessary?

Vitamins are chemicals your body needs (in very small amounts) to function properly. They are needed for the proper utilization of proteins, carbohydrates, fats, and other nutrients. Vitamins also help your body manufacture some of its vital substances, including red blood cells, hormones, and other chemicals. Since your body cannot make all the vitamins it needs, you must obtain some of them from the foods you eat.

The body also needs a certain amount of minerals. Minerals such as calcium, iron, phosphorus, magnesium, sodium, potassium, and zinc perform a variety of functions essential for your well-being. Calcium and phosphorus are essential for the growth of strong teeth and bones. Sodium (found in salt) is a major component of body fluid outside our cells, while potassium exists inside our cells. Deficiencies in these and other trace minerals can lead to serious problems because these chemicals help conduct small electrical impulses through nerves and muscles, allowing movement, coordination, and heart function.

Iron, of course, is important in the formation of the red blood cells (those that carry oxygen). Magnesium plays an important role in many essential chemical reactions (such as enzyme reactions). Zinc helps maintain tissue growth and improves the ability to heal after injury.

How can I know if my diet provides me with enough vitamins and minerals?

Your body needs only trace amounts of vitamins and minerals. These amounts, called *recommended daily allowances (RDA's),* thought to be enough to maintain normal health, are published by the Food and Nu-

27

trition Board for the National Academy of Sciences National Research Council. Your doctor may be able to give you a copy of the most recent RDA's, or you can find them at your local library.

If you are a healthy person who, each day, eats a variety of foods from the 4 basic food groups (2 milk products, 2 meat products, 4 vegetables/fruits, and 4 bread/cereal products), and who consumes over 1500 calories a day, it's unlikely that you lack any of the essential vitamin and mineral preparations.

Some processed foods are labeled to show you the vitamins and minerals they contain and the quantities of each.

Is there anyone who needs to take a daily multivitamin/ mineral pill?

As we've already discussed, if you are currently on a weight-loss diet, taking in less than 1500 calories a day, you probably do need to take a vitamin/mineral preparation. If you are pregnant or breast-feeding, it is possible, but difficult, to obtain the adequate amounts of vitamins and minerals you need through a proper diet. Many physicians prescribe a specially formulated multivitamin/mineral preparation for pregnant women or women who breast-feed to make sure they do not lack any of the vital nutrients.

If you are a vegetarian who eats no foods of animal origin, including milk products or eggs, you could become deficient in iron, calcium, vitamin B-12, and zinc. Vegetarians must carefully plan their diets to make sure that they get adequate amounts of these vitamins and minerals or that they are supplemented through the use of a multivitamin/mineral pill.

Finally, doctors also know that patients who are recovering from an operation or illness, even if they can eat a normal diet, have special needs in the vitamin/mineral group and may require a supplement.

EATING DISORDERS

What is anorexia nervosa?

As long as we are talking about nutrition and dieting, we should talk about 2 of the most extreme types of nutritional disorders. Anorexia nervosa is an illness involving self-starvation and an extreme aversion to food. It typically affects teenage women from the middle to upper-middle classes who are very bright, high achievers in school and are seemingly well adjusted. Most people with anorexia nervosa are white females, but about 6% are adolescent white males. Occasionally, the illness is seen in older women.

It has been estimated that 1 in 250 adolescent females has anorexia and that 1 in 25 American teenage girls experiences some anorexialike symptoms. The incidences of anorexia seem to be increasing, but the cause is unknown. Researchers can identify the psychological patterns associated with this disorder—anorexia is most often found in teenage girls who are high achievers and who strive for affection and approval. In our society where thinness is prized, the anorexic begins to diet. After losing a few pounds, the anorexic becomes obsessed with losing more, and soon an abnormal concern with weight loss and dieting is established.

The symptoms of anorexia nervosa are rapid weight loss, cessation of the menstrual cycle, and a range of behavior patterns, such as compulsive and excessive exercise, related to the individual's fear of being fat. In extreme cases, physical symptoms such as hair loss, severe constipation, intolerance to cold temperatures, and slow pulse rate result. Often an anorexic teenager will withdraw from society. He or she will become so compulsive about avoiding food that the young person simply will not eat at all.

Treatment for anorexia nervosa involves treatment of the individual's nutritional problem and intensive psychotherapy and family counseling. If the weight loss is severe, the person may need to be hospitalized. Approximately 10% to 20% of anorexics die as a result of their illness.

What is bulimia?

The other extreme eating disorder is bulimia. People with bulimia eat large amounts of food and then induce vomiting to ensure that they will not gain weight. Sometimes bulimics will use strong laxatives to purge their systems of all the food they take in. Unlike anorexics, bulimics tend to have normal body weight, but their eating behavior is secretive and destructive. The constant loss of gastric juices, vitamins, and minerals from the system because of the vomiting and purging can cause serious potassium deficiencies and other medical problems. Bulimia affects a wide age range, occurring in teenage girls as well as in older women. As with anorexia, the treatment of bulimia is intensive nutritional therapy and psychological counseling.

EXERCISE

Why is it important to exercise?

Regular exercise is essential to good health for everybody. It strengthens the heart and other muscles, improves circulation, protects against brittle bones and adult-onset diabetes, aids in weight loss, relieves stress, and restores stamina and energy. If we consider the multiple benefits of exercise, it would seem that all Americans would be exercising. However, study after study shows us that a large percentage of the population does no regular exercise. There are probably a lot of reasons for this, many related to our advanced technology. Not many of us have to do hard, physical labor any more. A great many people have sedentary jobs, and the only walking they may do is to the water cooler or the coffee machine.

You can imagine what would happen to your finely tuned, expensive automobile if you let it sit in the garage, day after day and year after year. If you suddenly decided to drive this neglected car on a long trip, you'd quickly find that it was unable to meet the demands placed upon it. Your body is the same way; it needs regular use—exercise—to function properly. Your heart needs the stimulation of regular exercise to maintain its strength.

Who should exercise?

People of all ages should get some form of exercise. We all know the importance of exercise in young people to maintain proper growth and muscle tone. However, as we grow older, exercise is equally important. The surgeon general tells us that exercise is a critical component for good health.

Routine exercise programs should be part of our daily lives. Young children need exercise to maintain good growth and development of bones and muscles. Teenagers need exercise to maintain good development of muscles and bones, especially during growth spurts. Young adults should exercise to improve their overall health and also their sense of well-being during that critical stage when most are beginning careers. During this time, we form our good health habits that will be carried on through later life. Young adults in the 20 to 30 age group who do not begin a regular exercise program generally will not change their exercise habits as they get older.

People who have reached their early 30's should be concerned about getting regular exercise as a prevention against heart disease in later years. Regular exercise is a major contributor to a strong, healthy heart.

You're never too old to begin an exercise program. If you have never exercised and are over 40 years of age, it's certainly time to begin. Do realize, however, that you have to be a little more cautious about beginning an exercise program as you get older.

George Burns once said that people who act old tend to get old. I strongly recommend that people in their 60's or even 70's who do not follow a regular exercise program begin some form of exercise to maintain good health and a sense of well-being. Of course, the type of exercise you do in your 60's or 70's will probably be somewhat different from what you do in your 30's. But that doesn't mean that you can't exercise.

When should I see my doctor if I'm going to begin an exercise program?

Certain people should consult their physician before beginning a regular exercise program. If you are under 40, in good health, and have no underlying health problems, then you can probably begin an exercise program as long as you use good sense. Begin the exercise program very slowly, and take 4 to 6 weeks to build up gradually to the level of exercise you would like to maintain.

If you are over 40, have high blood pressure, heart disease, diabetes, or have a family history of any of these diseases, check with your physician before beginning a regular exercise program. No matter what your age, if you are more than 25 to 30 pounds overweight, you should check with your doctor. Any special health problems create a need to tailor the type of exercise program you begin. This doesn't mean that you can't begin an exercise program, it simply means that you need to check with your physician so that together you can work out a *proper* exercise plan for your special needs.

What is the best exercise to do?

The best exercise is the kind you enjoy and will continue doing on a regular basis. For some people this means bicycling; for others, it means swimming; for a large portion of the population, it means jogging. Doctors can't say that a particular type of exercise is better than another in terms of health benefits—a person who jogs does not necessarily get more benefits than someone who is on a good bicycling program. The key to choosing your type of exercise is to find something you enjoy. If you enjoy it you'll stick with it. If you don't, you'll quickly drop the program. Do you know someone who began a jogging program but detested it or actually had discomfort from it? How long do you think a program like that really lasted? It probably ended the 1st time it rained or a knee began to ache.

A good form of exercise that almost anyone can do, regardless of age and most physical problems, is walking. Walking is excellent exercise, and if tailored to the individual's age and health, it can result in maximum health benefits.

I actually write prescriptions for walking programs to give patients who need to lose weight, increase cardiovascular stamina, or simply relieve stress. It's quite simple. I tell them to go out in their automobile and map out a mile around their home. I then instruct them to begin walking 1 mile every evening for approximately 2 weeks. During those 1st weeks, they walk the mile in about 15 to 20 minutes. At the end of the 1st 2 weeks, I ask them to increase their speed, so that they finish the mile in 12 or 15 minutes. Then the patients begin to increase the distance up to 2 miles. Over the next month, they begin walking 2 miles every night and get to the point where they can walk those 2 miles in 20 to 25 minutes. For some people, this will be extremely slow, but for a person 60 to 65 years old, with some degree of arthritis in the legs, this can be a very fast clip.

I do regular exercise, but I get so many aches and pains.

Most of the muscle aches and pains you get through regular exercise are due to failure to do the proper amount of warm-up exercises prior to beginning the exercise program. Muscles are tight fibers that will respond with pain when stretched beyond their normal use. If you simply get up from behind your desk some evening and go out and walk a mile or so without any kind of warm-up, then your muscles will probably respond with pain, aching, and perhaps even swelling. Therefore, it is important to spend 10 to 15 minutes before you begin your exercise program doing some stretching exercises to relieve the tension and tightness in your muscles.

Most stretching exercises involve the legs and the upper extremities. Simply going up on your toes and back down to your heels for about 2 or 3 minutes will stretch the calf muscles and the hamstrings, the muscles in the back of the leg. Another good exercise is to lean toward a wall or a parked car and stretch backward with 1 foot so that only the toe meets the ground, then stretch forward to loosen your calves. You will push backward, stretch and then relax, push forward, stretch and then relax. This is important, especially before jogging, to limber up the calves and the Achilles tendons.

In your warm-up exercises, don't forget to stretch the upper body by gently twisting from side to side and rotating the shoulders.

Something that even the most avid exercisers seem to forget is the cool-down exercise. If you have walked for a couple of miles or jogged 10 miles, you are hot and sweaty and your muscles are tired when you get back. If you immediately go indoors, especially into an air-conditioned room, and flop down, you'll find that the next time you go out and jog you'll have lots of tenderness, tightness, and pain in your muscles. When you get back home, make sure that you repeat the same stretching exercises you did earlier, allowing your muscles to relax and cool down.

Can I do regular exercise if I have arthritis?

Even people with severe arthritis can exercise. Arthritis can be devastating, both physically and psychologically, but exercise can help many arthritics win back some freedom of movement and with it a sense of independence and self-confidence. The benefits of a carefully managed exercise program for an arthritic are a reduction in the muscle shortening and joint contractions, fewer muscle spasms, improved circulation, an increased range of motion, and a decreased likelihood of deformities in the future.

If you have arthritis and are going to begin an exercise program, make sure you check with your physician. Here are some pointers:
• Do not exercise beyond the point of pain.
• Never exercise if you have hot, inflamed joints.
• Do not stay in 1 position for more than 20 minutes at a time; shift positions frequently.
• Don't overdo it—cut down on how much you squeeze into each day, like work, social life, recreation, or other commitments.
• Rest when you feel tired.
• Never exercise when you are the stiffest, such as in the morning.
• Exercise each arthritic joint at least once a day.
• Make sure that all of your exercise movements are slow and gradual. And check with your local arthritis foundation for some helpful literature on how to begin an exercise program when you have arthritis.

Can I exercise if I've had a heart attack?

Years ago anyone who had a heart attack was generally considered to be almost totally disabled for the rest of his life. However, over the past several years, we have begun to understand the extreme importance of getting people who have had a heart attack on a regular exercise program. Of course, the type of program depends upon your age and the seriousness of your heart disease, but the vast majority of people (especially ages 40 to 65) who have had heart attacks can and should begin a supervised exercise program.

Heart rehabilitation centers have sprung up all over the country. In these centers, qualified physicians work with heart patients in devising proper exercise programs to increase heart capacities and improve chances against further heart disease.

What does my heart rate have to do with my exercise program?

An efficient way to figure out whether you are doing too much or too little exercise is to monitor your maximum heart or pulse rate. When your physician evaluates your exercise program, he or she will give you certain parameters as a guide to how fast your heart races while you are exercising. A more sophisticated way to do this is to place you on a treadmill machine and find out how fast your heart beats during controlled exercise. An easier way to do it is to simply subtract your age from 220. If you are 50 years old, subtracting 50 from 220 is 170. The maximum heart rate, or target pulse, that you should achieve or maintain during strenuous exercise should be approximately 70% of that number, or 120. When you exercise, stop periodically and take your pulse for 15 seconds and multiply that number by 4. If your heart rate is close to the desired 70% rate, then you are achieving good cardiovascular exercise.

Can I achieve a regular exercise program if I am a diabetic?

The American Diabetes Association states that exercise is just as important as diet in the management of both major types of diabetics— those who require insulin and those who are controlled either with diet or with oral medication. Exercise makes a diabetic's cells more sensitive to insulin. Thus, exercise reduces the external insulin requirements for insulin-dependent diabetics and also enhances the blood glucose control for those who are not dependent upon insulin.

Any diabetic needs to understand the changes that occur and the precautions needed before beginning a regular exercise program. An exercise program will increase the number of calories burned during the exercise; therefore, diabetics on a regular exercise program will need to increase their daily caloric intake to account for their routine exercise program. Diabetics who take insulin injections need to carefully watch their blood sugar and urine sugar levels. Proper adjustments of both insulin and caloric intake can allow any diabetic to maintain an active exercise program.

What is aerobic training?

The basic goal of most exercise programs is to increase the body's capacity to capture the oxygen from the air and to transport that oxygen to all the cells of the body. Most of us are able to capture enough oxygen for ordinary use. Otherwise we would be huffing and puffing all the time. Aerobic exercises make you huff and puff heavily; instead of just working your biceps or your waistline, aerobic exercises work your heart and lungs. Thus, the heart becomes stronger, the lungs become more efficient, and the cells get oxygen more easily. Once you build a reserve capacity, when your body needs extra oxygen your heart and lungs can supply it without a lot of huffing and puffing.

Should young people be placed on an exercise program?

It is important for children to avoid extremes. Children, no matter what age, should get the proper amount of exercise. But going to extremes can be potentially harmful for any child. No one knows exactly how much exercise a child can perform safely. Young children who are placed on vigorous exercise programs, such as marathon distance running, can suffer permanent muscle and bone damage. Children can suffer heel cord or bone injuries and are more prone to extreme temperature problems such as hypo- or hyperthermia. Dehydration, which causes the deaths of many young football players each year, must be guarded against, also.

Basically, children should be able to choose sports or activities that *they* like. Children should be allowed to drop an activity when they lose interest. Making kids do something that they don't enjoy can backfire by creating a long-standing hatred of a particular physical activity (that the child might resume if simply left alone). At the very least, children should get a minimum of 1 to 1½ hours of activity a day, by walking, bicycling, or just playing.

What are some specific types of exercise, and how should they be done?

There are several excellent types of exercise—all have basically equal value:

Walking. A brisk nonstop walk can get you in good shape if you do it for at least 45 to 60 minutes, 3 to 5 times a week.

Jogging. Alternate walking and jogging in 1 minute intervals until you can jog for at least 20 minutes at a time. To limit leg, foot, and knee injuries, always use the highest quality running shoes and avoid jogging on pavement.

Stationary cycling. Stationary cycling generally causes fewer injuries than jogging and can be done at home in any weather. This is a very good choice for both elderly and overweight people.

Swimming. Swimming is an excellent form of exercise, although obviously not available to everyone. Swimming causes no stress on joints and offers resistance to muscles without straining them. To get the maximum benefits from swimming, do long, slow laps. Because water lessens the pull of gravity, your target pulse would probably be 10 to 15 points lower than the 70% figure we calculated earlier.

Other activities can be very beneficial for your exercise program: *hiking, rowing, skiing, aerobic dancing,* and *aerobic exercises* are all good if they are done vigorously for approximately 1 hour. Exercises such as *tennis* and *golf* are also good but don't keep you quite as active for long enough periods of time to have maximum cardiovascular benefit. Playing golf is *not* an exercise when you ride a cart for 18 holes. If you are trying to achieve a good exercise program and combine it with your golf game, make sure (if you are physically able) that you walk the 18 holes and carry your bag.

SMOKING

Is smoking really bad for you?

The American Medical Association, the American Heart Association, the American Cancer Society, and the surgeon general of the United States all unanimously agree that smoking is bad for you. According to the American Cancer Society, almost 500,000 Americans each year die prematurely from diseases that are directly related to smoking: heart disease, stroke, and cancer are the leading causes of death in this country. Cigarette smoking is a major cause of lung cancer, emphysema, heart disease, and chronic bronchitis. Smoking is strongly linked with certain cancers, especially cancer of the larynx (the voice box), the mouth, the esophagus, and the urinary bladder. Smoking has also been shown to be associated with an increased risk of stroke and other circulatory disease.

The health hazards related to smoking are directly proportional to the number of cigarettes you smoke per day. The earlier the age at which you started smoking and the longer you continue to smoke, the greater your risk of developing serious health problems.

Smoke contains hundreds of chemical substances including nicotine, tar, and carbon monoxide. Nicotine causes the blood vessels to constrict or tighten, which in turn forces the heart to pump faster and faster, increasing the stress on the cardiovascular system.

Very tiny particles of tar settle on the membranes of your breathing passages and destroy normal lung tissue. Tar also contains chemicals that have produced cancer in experimental animals.

Carbon monoxide reduces the oxygen-carrying ability of your normal red blood cells. If you smoke, as much as 10% of the oxygen that would normally be carried by your red blood cells is driven out by the carbon monoxide. That means even in the best of circumstances, someone who smokes is walking around with only 90% of the oxygen required.

The risk of death from lung cancer is 10 times greater for the average male smoker than for the nonsmoker, according to the American Cancer Society. The risk of death from heart disease is also 4 to 5 times greater for the smoker.

I might note that the lung cancer and heart disease death rate for females used to be relatively low. But over the last 20 years, the number of females suffering from these kinds of cancer, heart disease, and stroke has increased. Most feel that this is directly related to the increased incidence of female smokers.

Is smoking really bad for you? The question has to be answered with an unequivocal yes. Cigarette smoking is dangerous.

If I have been smoking for years, will it do me any good to stop?

No matter how long you've smoked, it pays to stop. Even after you have smoked 20 or 40 years, your body starts to recover from the effects of smoking as soon as you quit. For example, your chances of developing lung cancer are dramatically reduced 5 years after you have stopped smoking. The chance of heart disease drops sharply within the 1st year after quitting. Within 10 years the ex-smoker's risk of heart disease is about the same as that of a nonsmoker.

People who have smoked for a long time tend to use the excuse, "Well, I have already damaged myself so I might as well continue to smoke." I must emphasize that people who stop smoking get positive benefits. If you smoke and develop a severe lung disease like emphysema, quitting may not make you dramatically better, but it certainly won't make you worse.

I've heard a lot about the positive effects of smoking. Are these just myths?

People who smoke use a lot of excuses to continue to smoke. They talk about the positive effects that smoking has on them. Of course, none of them will talk about the risk factors of developing heart disease, cancer, or lung disease. Many people say that smoking is relaxing and, therefore, reduces the stress in their lives. But smoking cigarettes actually increases rather than decreases the tension level in your body. The reason for this is that nicotine, the primary chemical in tobacco, affects the sympathetic nervous system and causes the release of a chemical called adrenalin, a hormone associated with feelings of stress and nervousness.

37

Other smokers talk about the fact that cigarettes help their ability to concentrate. Adequate concentration is based on an adequate supply of oxygen to all the cells, especially those of the brain. When you consider the fact that if you are a smoker, a good deal of your oxygen is being replaced by carbon monoxide, then you see that you have less oxygen available and a decreased ability to concentrate.

Another myth is that smoking helps to control your weight. Experiments at the American Health Foundation suggest that while some people do gain weight after quitting, others stay the same and many even lose weight. The fact is, your weight can be controlled. The hazardous effects of even a 15 to 20 pound weight gain after stopping smoking is certainly less than the health hazards of continuing the nicotine habit.

If I stop smoking, how can I control my weight?

People are almost as obsessed with weight gain as they are with cigarette smoking. However, a very practical approach to your weight during the period of stopping smoking can significantly control your weight gain.

It is important for people who are preparing to stop smoking to also place themselves on an appropriate diet during this period. A basic fundamental of a good diet says that you don't skip meals. Research again indicates that many people who smoke tend to skip meals and "have a cigarette" in place of it. If you are going to stop smoking make sure that you do not skip meals; eat 3 well-balanced meals a day. Make sure you eliminate foods that contain sugar as well as all alcoholic beverages. It's obvious that sugar contains calories, but people forget that substituting drinking for cigarette smoking can not only lead to potential problems with alcohol, it significantly increases the number of calories taken in.

A good dietary program also includes good eating habits. *Eat only while seated.* People who eat "on the run" eat more and eat more quickly—and most of the calories will turn into fat. Take at least 20 minutes to sit down and have a meal. This allows your brain to receive signals of fullness from your stomach. When you feel full, stop eating; don't continue eating because everyone else is.

Keep a daily record of the amount of food you consume in order to become more aware of what your eating patterns are. An eating record is extremely helpful to point out the types of foods you eat that could be contributing to your weight gain.

Never undertake a major weight-control effort when you're trying to stop smoking. It's stressful enough to stop smoking. Adding the stress of a weight-control program can be too much.

Can the new nicotine gum really help you stop smoking?

Studies by the American Lung Association show that 1 reason people have a difficult time stopping smoking is that there is actually a physical dependence on the chemical nicotine. But there is another side to the problem—the psychological addiction to the mechanics of smoking.

An effective approach to ceasing the tobacco habit is to work with the physical dependence on the chemical nicotine while utilizing techniques to break the psychological habit. A chewing gum that contains nicotine releases small amounts of nicotine over a period of time to satisfy the physical craving. Once that takes place, you can focus on a technique or follow an accepted program to break the psychological dependence on the mechanics of smoking.

A word of caution: Nicotine gum is *not* a cure. People who are not motivated to stop smoking will not stop, regardless of the amount of gum they use. This is a new medication that can help you give up cigarettes, and it is designed as a temporary aid to help reduce the effects of withdrawing from nicotine. The nicotine gum cannot accomplish the job alone. You need a lot of willpower to break a habit as strong as cigarette smoking.

What is the best way to quit smoking?

There are as many different types of smokers as there are people who smoke, so there is not 1 program that will help everybody. But there are some indicators that can point out whether or not someone is going to be successful.

We know that people must be motivated to be successful. This sounds like a very simple statement, but a lot of people will say they "want to quit" when deep down they would really like to continue smoking. This conflict produces a lack of dedication to accomplishing the goal.

The vast majority of people who stop the cigarette habit (and remain stopped) do so by going "cold turkey." Others substitute 1 brand for another, smoking a low-nicotine cigarette instead of a high-nicotine cigarette, or change from a regular cigarette to menthol to break the cycle of the habit. However, at some point in time, a person who is motivated to stop smoking will simply have to take the package out of pocket or purse, throw it away, and never touch another cigarette.

Something that seems to work with most people is preparing to quit smoking. Smokers who have not really thought about stopping but who, after a bad coughing spell, say to themselves, "I'm never going to

39

touch another cigarette," have not truly prepared themselves for that red-letter day. Their success rate is not usually good. I recommend that you actually psyche yourself up and pick a certain day some time in the future to be the day when you will not smoke any more.

I also strongly recommend that you read the literature put out by the American Cancer Society. These are very good hints that most people can follow on their own if, in fact, they are truly motivated.

DRINKING

Is drinking harmful to your health?

It has been said that if alcohol were just being introduced to our country, it would probably never be approved for sale because of its harmful effects upon the body. Alcohol is a chemical that is quickly transferred to almost all tissues as soon as it is taken into the body. Most of the effects we notice relate to its action upon the brain, but alcohol is also immediately taken up in other organs such as the liver, heart, stomach, and kidneys.

When alcohol is swallowed, it is absorbed rapidly through the stomach and wall of the small intestine. This rapid absorption causes an almost immediate elevation in the amount of alcohol in the blood, commonly referred to as the blood alcohol. Once alcohol is in the bloodstream, it is rapidly distributed throughout the body and carried to the brain, where it influences behavior.

Some of the more notable changes are lessened alertness, decreased reaction time, and impaired judgment. These effects can be seen within the first hour after taking even 1 alcoholic drink.

While this is taking place within the brain, the alcohol is also being distributed to other parts of the body, such as the liver, which has a hard time metabolizing or handling the breakdown of alcohol; the liver itself can become damaged. The short-term and cumulative impact of alcohol on the body is significant.

It is estimated that billions of dollars are lost each year due to health problems and loss of work time related to alcohol.

Psychologically, many people use alcohol to calm down and relax, under the misconception that it will help them make better decisions. The ability to reason and make logical, intelligent judgments is markedly reduced when alcohol is consumed. We have all witnessed the emotional changes that take place when people drink. Short-term changes include depression and/or belligerence, but severe emotional problems can result from extended alcohol consumption.

Alcohol is a leading contributor to death in our country—just behind heart disease and cancer. Alcohol-related deaths due to automobile accidents and suicides increase year after year. Not only does the alcoholic suffer, but often the entire family unit is victimized as well. The emotional stress placed on the spouse and children by the alcoholic can be devastating.

How can I tell if I am developing alcoholism?

According to the American Psychiatric Association, a diagnosis of alcohol dependence is based upon how and why an individual uses alcohol, how that alcohol affects the home life and the job, and the ability of the person to stop drinking entirely.

Here are some of the characteristic patterns associated with the development of alcoholism:
- Having to use alcohol every day just to function properly
- The inability to stop drinking or even cut down on the amount that you drink
- Going on binges—remaining intoxicated throughout the day for at least 2 days at a time
- Two or more blackout spells that occur while you are drinking
- The inability to stop drinking despite the fact that you are developing serious physical problems

If any or all of these factors apply to you, there is a strong possibility that you are developing alcohol dependence or alcoholism.

Is alcoholism really an illness?

In the past, alcoholics were condemned and rejected. The alcoholic was stereotyped as the derelict or wino portrayed in the movies. However, health professionals have come to understand that alcoholism is a disease. Defining *alcoholism* as "significant impairment that is directly associated with persistent and excessive use of alcohol," the medical establishment now recognizes that alcoholism is a disease, not just a social problem.

As the attitude toward alcoholism has changed, innovative and progressive techniques of treatment have begun. Instead of being placed in a jail cell to "sober up" overnight, alcoholics are treated from a total medical approach utilizing current medical therapies, psychological counseling, and behavior modification.

How common is alcoholism?

Alcoholism is an extensive, progressive, and serious health problem. There is no accurate count of the number of alcoholics in the United States, but estimates range from 10 to 20 million, depending upon the definition used. In 1977, the President's Commission on Mental Health indicated that approximately 10 million Americans had a significant alcohol-related problem and that another 10 million either had or would suffer the same fate. The report further stated that out of this 20 million, close to 1 million were receiving help at that time.

Whatever the incidence of alcoholism, no one can doubt its serious medical, social, and economic consequences. The cost to our nation is estimated at $25 billion a year from job absenteeism, health and welfare programs, and medical expenses. Moreover, figures from the National Safety Council list alcohol as a factor in over ½ the fatal automobile crashes and adult pedestrian accidents.

How much is too much?

The National Institute of Alcohol Abuse and Alcoholism warns that drinking in moderation may not be universally harmful but that we don't know which people are going to react to what level of alcohol. It simply is not possible to know how much is too much for each individual. Compounding the problem is the fact that moderation is often haphazardly defined. What constitutes moderation for 1 person may be an excess for another.

There is no way to specify a safe limit, but we can define a *heavy drinker* as a "person who averages 2 drinks or more a day." A standard drink is 14 grams of pure alcohol, which is approximately 1½ ounces of 80 proof spirits, 5 ounces of 12% table wine, or 13 ounces of 4.5% beer.

Using these strict guidelines, most American drinkers have crossed over the boundary. At last report, national consumption was more than 300 million gallons of alcohol a year—an average of 3 drinks a day for some 110 million people.

Are alcoholics always adults?

The National Institute of Alcohol Abuse and Alcoholism estimates that perhaps 4 to 5 million young people have significant drinking problems. The extent of alcoholism among America's teenagers is alarming, and it is increasing rapidly. A casual beer in the backseat of a car used to be exciting for a teenager, but now many have a drinking problem that requires 2 or more drinks per day while at school. Teenagers hide liquor bottles in school lockers and drink between classes. Increasing numbers drive while under the influence of alcohol; teenage deaths in alcohol-related automobile accidents is rapidly increasing. Alcoholism is a disease that affects all ages—young and old.

How can I quit drinking?

The 1st step in stopping is admitting that you have a drinking problem. Alcoholics Anonymous will tell you that the most important statement a problem drinker can make is to freely admit "I am an alcoholic."

Once a problem drinker admits that he or she is an alcoholic, the next step is to seek help. Studies have shown that it is almost impossible for people to change on their own; they need the help and support of groups that are familiar with the techniques needed to stop drinking. Anyone who answers "yes" to the questions about problem drinking should call Alcoholics Anonymous, a local support group for alcoholics, or a physician. Just as in stopping smoking, the most important step is wanting to stop. Once that decision is made, help can be obtained through an experienced therapist who uses a medical approach for the disease of alcoholism and a psychological approach for the psychological addiction.

STRESS

What is stress?

Stress is an internal feeling that results when our expectations in life far exceed our achievements. The gap between expectation and achievement in the real world results in the internal turmoil we call stress.

If this gap between expectation and achievement is too wide, people feel such pressure to achieve that they mobilize tremendous amounts of energy and then have no way to release it. This creates a feeling of frustration and the unused energy turns inward, creating psychological and emotional problems. Approximately ⅔ of all office visits to family physicians in this country are related to unrelieved stress and its effects on mind and body.

Untreated stress can result in an increased incidence of heart disease, high blood pressure, and other physical illness. We all need to recognize the problem of stress and learn more innovative ways to cope with it.

How can we control stress in our lives?

43

There are some very good techniques we can use to deal with stress. No technique is going to take away all the stress of our jobs or our personal lives, but it can allow us to handle stress better.

The 1st step you should take if you are under a tremendous amount of stress is to try to get control of your life. Remember, stress is the difference between what you expect of yourself and what you actually achieve. When this miscalculation occurs, life begins to control you rather than the other way around. A simple but effective technique is to select a single aspect of your life that you would like to improve, write it down, and learn different ways to make gains in this area. For example, you may choose the area of education and begin to concentrate on ways to become better educated. During this initial phase, all the other complications of your life will take a backseat to this new focus.

Another important point in dealing with stress is to set realistic goals for yourself. Most of us go by the old adage that we should always set our sights a little higher than we can really reach. However, when we do this too often, the result is stress. Make sure the goals you set for yourself in sports, business, or your personal life are realistic and obtainable. When you obtain 1 goal, set another for yourself.

It's been said that we should all act as though we had only 6 months to live—doing only the things we have to do, accomplishing only the things we have to accomplish, and eliminating the rest.

Anybody in a stressful situation needs to strike a balance between work and play. All work and no play makes anyone dull and stressful.

These few simple tips will help you deal better with stress. They won't take away the stressful situations of a family crisis, economic problems, or a job situation you don't like. But they will help you adjust to the stress, and this adjustment is the critical issue.

How does stress influence my health?

To understand the effects of stress on your health, you need to think about a previous stressful situation. Let's say you became angry on the job. You lost your temper and pounded your fist on the table. What did you feel? Well, you probably felt your heart racing a little faster, your blood pressure went up, your muscles felt tense and achy, and your circulation shut down, making your extremities cold or tingly. All of these changes in your body are connected with the release of a chemical called adrenalin. Adrenalin, released in periods of stress, causes an immediate response throughout the body, especially your cardiovascular system.

The release of adrenalin is very helpful during periods of stress or danger when you need immediate energy. But if this goes on time after time, the positive effects are gone and the negative results of stress set in.

People under stress have an increased risk of developing high blood pressure, heart attacks, stomach ulcers, tension headaches, and many other health problems. Stress is probably an underlying factor in the development of many serious and life-threatening illnesses.

Is exercise good for stress?

A positive benefit of exercise is the reduction of stress within our lives. In fact, I strongly advise my patients who are under a great deal of stress to begin a routine exercise program. It is good for overall health, and seems to significantly reduce the effects stress has on the body.

The same types of exercise that improve the cardiovascular system can be used to reduce stress. A nightly walk or jog can significantly relieve the tensions of the day. It can also improve sleep patterns, and the better a person sleeps, the better he or she will be able to get up and cope with the pressures of the next day.

OTHER ISSUES LEADING TO GOOD HEALTH

How can seat belts be considered a factor in good health?

Each year thousands of Americans are killed in automobile accidents. If we were talking about some form of disease and said that thousands of Americans died from a disease that could have been prevented if the patient had only known about the cure, then we would all get up in arms and demand that the public be told about the cure. Well, thousands of Americans die each year in automobile accidents, usually within 5 to 10 miles from home, because they did not wear their seat belts. If we are going to discuss health factors such as diet, exercise, and stress reduction, then we must emphasize the importance of preventable deaths in automobile accidents. Every person who gets into a car without buckling the seat belt is playing Russian roulette.

Why all the emphasis on child safety seats?

According to the Insurance Institute for Highway Safety, about 650 children under the age of 5 are killed in automobile wrecks in the United States each year. Most of these deaths could have been prevented if the children were placed in properly-fitted infant or toddler safety seats or restrained with a seat belt.

How many times have you seen an adult get into a car, strap the seat belt, and let children in the backseat crawl all over each other or stand up on the seat?

It is the responsibility of every adult who drives a car to make sure that every other adult fastens the seat belt and that every child in the car is either strapped in with a seat belt or is sitting in a properly-fitted child safety seat.

IMPORTANT LIFE-SAVING PROCEDURES

What is CPR?

Suppose I tell you that you could save a life without ever going to medical school or getting a nursing degree. What would you say? Well, every day in our country, thousands of lives are saved because you, the average citizen, know how to respond in an emergency situation such as an acute heart attack. The American Heart Association estimates that 50% of people who suffer acute heart attacks die before reaching the hospital; many of these people could be saved.

Cardiopulmonary resuscitation (CPR) techniques are used to effectively treat acute heart attacks and other catastrophic events, such as electrocution and drowning. CPR is a combination of techniques that can be implemented by *anyone* to maintain the heart rate and breathing of the victim until qualified medical specialists are available.

Everyone should learn CPR. Young children can learn it. Older people can learn it. The rest of us can, too. CPR classes are given by hospitals, physician organizations, the American Heart Association, American Red Cross, and many other civic groups. Next time this course is given, join up. You may save a life.

How can I help someone who is choking on a piece of food?

This is another life-threatening situation that needs immediate attention. If a piece of food is trapped at the opening of the windpipe, a person cannot breathe. If you see someone eating a meal, then grab the throat and have difficulty breathing, the person could be choking. Another clue is if the person has difficulty speaking. Both of these are symptoms of choking and if breathing is not restored in a few minutes, that person will die. However, if you know a simple technique called the *Heimlich maneuver,* you can save a life.

The principle of the Heimlich maneuver is to forcefully and suddenly increase the pressure in the upper abdomen, enough to push the lodged particles back up through the throat and out the mouth. When you see someone choking, immediately follow these steps:

46

1. Position yourself behind the victim.
2. Place your arms around the victim, clasping your hands, palms down, in the middle of the victim's stomach just below the ribs.
3. Then, with a quick, forceful movement, thrust inward and slightly upward into the victim's stomach.
4. Repeat the move several times until the food particle has cleared or further help arrives.

Heimlich maneuver techniques should be learned by everyone. They are usually posted in restaurants, but what about at home? What would happen if a friend or family member were to begin to choke? Would you know what to do? Learn the Heimlich maneuver—before you need it.

2.

A Healthy Pregnancy
Leads to a Healthy Baby

PREGNANCY TESTS AND PRENATAL CARE

How can I tell if I am pregnant?

A lot of women tell me that they simply "know" when they are pregnant—they have a feeling or sense that their whole body has changed. Traditionally, however, the diagnosis of pregnancy is made when a woman has missed 1 or more periods. Of course, many women will occasionally skip a period, and that doesn't mean they are pregnant. Usually physicians don't become concerned until a woman has missed her 2nd period. By that time, a woman may also have other signs of pregnancy, such as breast tenderness, frequent urination, or some early morning nausea. If you suspect you are pregnant, the pregnancy can be confirmed in 1 of 2 ways. The simplest method is to test the urine. Substances called estradiol are produced in a woman during pregnancy, and the urine test can generally detect a pregnancy 3 to 4 weeks after conception.

Of course, a lot of women want to know if they are pregnant sooner than 3 or 4 weeks. If this is the case, a serum pregnancy test can be ordered immediately upon missing your 1st period. This particular test looks for the presence of estradiol in your blood and is so sensitive it may show if you're pregnant within 10 days to 2 weeks after conception.

Many test kits for pregnancy are now available in drugstores. These urine tests, although not as sensitive, also measure the estradiol in the urine.

48

Once I find out that I am pregnant, what should I do next?

As soon as you find out that you are pregnant, you should consult your physician or obstetrician. Whether your doctor is a family physician who delivers babies or an obstetrician, he or she will set up a series of prenatal visits to the office. The responsibility of the physician who will be delivering your baby is to ensure that you, the mother, stay healthy throughout the 9 months of pregnancy. These prenatal visits are also crucial to the ultimate health of your unborn child. Studies by the U.S. Department of Health, Education, and Welfare in the early 1970s and by the American Academy of Pediatrics show that women who get into prenatal care early in the pregnancy are more likely to have healthier pregnancies and, therefore, healthier children than women who neglect such care. During these visits, your physician will test you for a series of medical problems that, if present, could complicate your pregnancy. He or she will make sure that your blood pressure stays normal, that your blood sugar does not show the presence of diabetes, and that your weight remains normal. You will also get started on some prenatal vitamins to ensure adequate nutrition for you and your unborn child.

How often will I need to see my doctor during my pregnancy?

Most prenatal visits are scheduled routinely throughout the pregnancy. During the 1st trimester (the 1st 3 months of the pregnancy), you will see your doctor approximately once a month. If your weight, blood pressure, and other tests remain normal during the 1st trimester, your doctor may elect to continue to see you monthly during the 2nd trimester. If complications are present, the physician will, of course, see you more often. During the last trimester, as your child begins to grow rapidly and your delivery date draws closer, most obstetricians and family physicians will schedule more frequent visits. The routine would be to see you every 2 weeks during the 7th and 8th months and about every week during the last month of your pregnancy. Again, I cannot overemphasize how important it is to maintain these frequent prenatal visits with your physician.

How important is my weight during my pregnancy?

Next to the health and well-being of the unborn baby, mothers tend to worry most about their own weight. Some will eat too much and know that they are eating too much, but don't seem to be able to stop. Others, in an effort to keep their weight gain to a minimum during pregnancy, don't eat nearly enough.

49

The old adage that "I'm eating for 2" is true, but it gets a lot of pregnant women into trouble. Today, most experts agree that the pregnant woman of normal weight should gain approximately 24 to 27 pounds during her pregnancy.

But, you ask, if the baby weighs only 6 to 8 pounds, why should I gain all that extra weight? Well, even though the unborn child may weigh only 6 to 8 pounds, a good deal of the rest of the weight is essential: the uterus itself weighs 2 pounds; the placenta about 1½ pounds; the combined amniotic fluid about 2 pounds; and the increased blood necessary for the child another 3 to 4 pounds. It's also important that the mother has stored fat and protein for the nourishment of the unborn child; this weighs approximately 4 pounds. Most mothers will also retain some fluid during their pregnancy, which adds up to about another 4 pounds. You can see that all of this "extra weight" is accounted for.

Is it all necessary? Absolutely. It is extremely important that the mother gain an adequate amount of weight and that it is distributed as shown above. You're not fat, you're pregnant. And the majority of that poundage will come off when the baby is born.

How should my weight gain be distributed during pregnancy?

During the 1st 3 months of pregnancy, you should probably count on gaining about 3 to 6 pounds. By the beginning of the 3rd month, weight gain should increase to about ¾ pound per week—about 1 pound every 9 days. By the middle of your pregnancy, you should have a weight gain of approximately 8 to 11 pounds. A weight gain of more than this is a warning sign to monitor your food intake. An unusually high weight gain could also signal the onset of swelling or edema, which requires immediate medical attention.

During the last trimester of pregnancy, the last 10 to 12 pounds will be added. A lot of this weight is added straight to the baby's weight. And remember, even though you're gaining weight, your baby definitely needs the vital nutrients you supply through your well-balanced diet.

What kind of diet should I eat if I get pregnant?

Once you find out that there is a baby on the way, you will want to be extra careful about what you eat. We know that about 80,000 calories are needed to produce a full-term baby, but you have to remember that those 80,000 calories are to be consumed over a 9-month period of time. A good guideline is that you should consume about 300 extra calories per day throughout the pregnancy, assuming that your activity level remains about the same as it did before you got pregnant. The added calories must supply energy, and all of the various nutrients required

50

for the unborn child. Without careful selection from the 4 basic food groups, it is easy to waste those 300 extra calories on a piece of chocolate cake or a candy bar that does not add any of the vitamins and minerals your baby really needs.

To help you calculate the approximate number of calories you will need during pregnancy, the National Academy of Sciences has developed a very simple method. Multiply your prepregnancy weight by 15, and then add 300. If your prepregnancy weight is about 120 pounds, you will require 120 times 15 (or 1800) calories plus 300, which equals 2100 total calories per day.

Remember that this is just a guideline. The more calories you burn, the more you will need to replace. If you are very active and continue to participate in sports or other strenuous activities during your pregnancy, the number of calories will obviously have to be raised.

Why does my doctor recommend vitamins and minerals during my pregnancy?

During pregnancy, additional amounts of vitamins from every category are needed, but folic acid, one of the B complex vitamins, is especially important. A pregnant woman requires twice as much folic acid as usual to avoid the risk of becoming anemic. Yeast, organ meats such as liver or kidney, and fresh green vegetables are all excellent natural sources of folic acid. Lesser amounts are also present in nearly all fresh foods. Since the need for folic acid escalates so dramatically during pregnancy, it is common for obstetricians or family physicians to prescribe vitamin B supplements.

The mother-to-be will also require additional amounts of niacin, thiamine (vitamin B-1), riboflavin (vitamin B-2), and vitamins B-6 and B-12. All are easily supplied through vitamin pills and protein-rich foods.

As far as minerals go, it is extremely important during pregnancy to increase the amount of calcium, iron, and zinc. The development of healthy bone structure in the unborn child is directly dependent upon an adequate supply of calcium in the mother's diet. About 50% more calcium than normal is required. During pregnancy the calcium that the mother takes in will shift directly to the baby, so if extra calcium is not added, the mother could develop brittle bones and teeth. Fortunately, two 8-ounce glasses of milk supply much of this needed calcium. Iron helps prevent anemia and assures the baby will develop adequate iron stores. Zinc assures proper metabolism of essential vitamins.

Why do some pregnant women need to take iron?

51

Pregnancy places increased demands on the amount of iron that women have within their systems. Remember that iron is utilized to create the blood cells that provide the vital nutrients and oxygen both to the woman and to the unborn child. Because of this increased demand on a woman's iron stores, most physicians will try to prevent any possibility of the woman's developing low iron by placing her on iron supplements.

To meet the normal requirements of pregnancy, all pregnant women should take supplemental vitamin and mineral capsules containing approximately 30 to 60 mg of elemental iron at least once a day. A woman whose iron level falls lower than expected should probably take prescription iron containing more than 30 to 60 mg. Remember that for best absorption, the iron supplement should be taken with orange juice 30 minutes before eating. If nausea results, the tablets may be taken with the midday or evening meal.

Can I take medications while I am pregnant?

Most physicians feel the fewer medications a woman takes during pregnancy, the better. This certainly doesn't mean that you can't take medication, but you should take it only for certain problems and only if prescribed by your physician. The problem with taking any medication during pregnancy centers on the effects that medication could have on the unborn child. Remember that during the first 3 months of pregnancy, major development of the child's organ systems is taking place. Therefore, medications taken during the 1st trimester can potentially have a more serious effect than the same medication taken later in the pregnancy. The best policy is not to take any medication during your pregnancy unless you have talked with your physician about it. If you need medication your physician will be able to select the right medication that has the least possibility of harm to you or to your unborn child.

And remember, if you are taking any medication at the time you find out that you are pregnant, be sure to tell your physician during your 1st prenatal visit.

ACTIVITIES DURING PREGNANCY

Can I continue to work if I am pregnant?

Many years ago it was common practice that once a woman became pregnant, she had to give up her job. This is no longer the case. In fact, active career women can maintain normal work loads during the first 7 to 8 months of pregnancy without any ill effects on the unborn child.

Many obstetricians and family physicians recommend that women continue to work because it keeps their exercise level up and makes the emotional adjustment to the pregnancy much easier. No woman should feel that if she gets pregnant she has to stop work, unless medical complications develop. If a woman's blood pressure rises too high or if the amount of swelling (edema) increases too dramatically, the physician may recommend she discontinue working for a while and rest at home until these conditions have been corrected.

Can I continue to exercise?

More and more women are jumping on the aerobic exercise bandwagon. Most pregnant women, even those in the 3rd trimester, can participate in this exercise program without jeopardizing the development of the unborn child.

A study conducted by an exercise physiologist at the University of Wisconsin showed that maternal exercise at about 70% of the maximum aerobic capacity increased the heart rate of the unborn child but did not affect the outcome of the pregnancy. These studies and others continue to show us that exercise can not only be continued—it is recommended.

A word of caution: always listen to your body. If you are exercising during your pregnancy and notice that you aren't feeling quite right, consult your physician immediately. Also any vaginal bleeding during exercise should be reported at once to your physician. If you exercise, be sure to wear supportive garments to avoid putting undue stress on already stretched ligaments. A good bra and a lightweight girdle should be worn during exercise.

What types of exercise are best during pregnancy?

Any exercise can be done by an otherwise healthy pregnant woman through the 1st 6 to 7 months of pregnancy. The further along a woman gets in her pregnancy, however, the more cautious she should be about the types of exercises she does. Strenuous exercises such as tennis, swimming, or jogging need to be cleared with a physician before continuing. However, almost all physicians will strongly recommend that women in the latter stages of pregnancy continue to do exercises that add strength and mobility to the abdomen and to the extremities.

Can I continue to enjoy sex during pregnancy?

This is a question most people want to ask, but they often are afraid to do so. Pregnancy is a major event for both the pregnant mother and the father. If it is the 1st pregnancy, there is often a tremendous concern or even fear that the pregnancy may result in an unhealthy child. In addition, many mothers- and fathers-to-be believe that sexual intercourse must stop during the pregnancy to avoid hurting or damaging the unborn child.

Many of the questions and problems regarding sexual intercourse during pregnancy stem from preexisting sexual relationships, not from the pregnancy itself. So, if there have been problems before pregnancy, the pregnancy will probably bring these problems to the forefront and create increasing difficulties. But if there has been a normal sexual relationship between the parents-to-be there is no reason why this relationship cannot continue.

Multiple studies show that there are no predictable changes in sexuality with pregnancy. During the 1st trimester, there is generally a great deal of breast enlargement, and some women will have trouble with nausea and vomiting because of increased estrogen levels, which stimulate changes in the uterus and continue to prepare the female body for a full-term pregnancy. As a result, there may be some interference in normal sexual patterns, but the nausea and vomiting usually pass fairly quickly. A lot of women also have an increased frequency of urination during the 1st part of the pregnancy, and this may interfere with, but should not significantly alter, normal sexual patterns.

The 2nd trimester is generally a stable period for the woman. The nausea has generally abated, and the urinary frequency is not as severe. During this time, sexual relations can be continued without any difficulty. It should be mentioned, however, that during this trimester many women will experience an increased desire for sexual attention, which needs to be understood by their husband. Where men generally get their sexual satisfaction through intercourse, during the 2nd trimester many women respond very positively to increased amounts of simple holding and touching.

The 3rd trimester, like the 1st, involves great changes. The fetus shows its greatest weight gain, and the woman's abdomen increases to a relatively large size. During this stage of the pregnancy, intercourse in the male superior position is neither possible nor comfortable. The couple may try a side-to-side position.

Numerous studies have appeared regarding the dangers of intercourse during the last stages of pregnancy. The most recent studies seem to indicate that there is no harm to the fetus as long as no medical complications to the pregnancy are present.

Pregnancy should be a happy time for both the father and the mother, and there is no reason that normal sexual relations cannot be continued throughout a healthy pregnancy.

HIGH-RISK PREGNANCY

What is meant by high-risk pregnancy?

Certain conditions may exist that can cause complications for a woman and thus place her pregnancy in the high-risk category. Some of these problems are hypertension, diabetes, or a previous history of complicated labor.

The reason it is so important to identify high-risk pregnancies is so special attention can be paid to the development of complications. If, for instance, a woman has diabetes and has had difficulties with her diabetes during previous pregnancies, then proper medications and/or insulin can be instituted to prevent these problems during the current pregnancy. If a woman has had a history of high blood pressure during a previous pregnancy, then sometimes adequate medications need to be instituted to prevent that blood pressure from getting out of control and endangering the unborn child.

Problems can also develop within the last trimester of pregnancy that can immediately place the pregnancy at risk. These include excessive fluid gain, an accelerated elevation of the blood pressure, and problems with the growth and development of the unborn child. If any of these are spotted during the last trimester of pregnancy, the physician will institute treatments to reduce the possibility that these complications could endanger the mother and the unborn child.

A primary reason that frequent prenatal visits are so strongly recommended is that early identification of a high-risk pregnancy can lead to more caution and specialized care during the pregnancy.

If I am in a high-risk category, how will my treatment change?

If you have, or develop, high-risk factors in your pregnancy, your physician will probably want to see you much more frequently. This way, he or she can evaluate any changes in the growth and development of the unborn child related to your particular risk factor. If, for instance, you are a diabetic, there is an increased chance that the physician will want to schedule an elected delivery at approximately 37 to 38 weeks. This early delivery is undertaken to decrease potential problems that the full-term (40-week) child could develop. Sometimes these early deliveries will be handled through a cesarean section, and the normal onset of labor will not be allowed to take place in order to protect the unborn child.

If your particular risk factor has to do with hypertension and if during the last trimester of pregnancy you develop a rather significant elevation of your blood pressure and/or fluid retention, your physician may recommend that you undergo strict bed rest and take proper medications. Some women's blood pressure and fluid retention increase so much during the last trimester that they actually have to be placed in the hospital for a period of time to control the situation.

All of these precautions sound scary, but if yours has been identified as a high-risk pregnancy, this does not mean that the outcome of the pregnancy cannot be a healthy baby. It simply means that it is very important for the physician to realize that you are in a high-risk category and to pay close attention to any potential developing complications. If you continue your frequent visits with your physician and if proper treatment is instituted early, then even high-risk category women such as diabetics and hypertensives can have normal, healthy pregnancies and normal, healthy children.

If I am a diabetic, should I still get pregnant?

As you know, diabetes occurs when a person's body can't handle sugar. Studies continue to show that a diabetic woman has the potential of more complications during pregnancy, and often may deliver a larger baby who has complications at birth related to the mother's diabetes. But remember that we've come a long way. Today we have sophisticated ways of treating diabetes, and physicians recognize the importance of controlling diabetes throughout the pregnancy.

Diabetics *can* get pregnant and *can* deliver healthy babies, however, these women are at risk and must be followed very closely. This may mean that the woman who was controlled by diet before her pregnancy may have to begin certain medications or even insulin to ensure a healthy newborn.

A lot of women will ask, "If I take insulin during my pregnancy will I have to continue the insulin after my child is born?" In the vast majority of cases, the answer is no. Once the pregnancy and its increased metabolic requirements are over, she can usually return to whatever treatment she was under prior to the pregnancy, provided that her weight also returns to normal. So, if a woman controlled her diabetes through simple diet before the pregnancy, after the pregnancy she should be able to do the same.

EFFECTS OF DRINKING AND SMOKING

What effect does alcohol have on the unborn child?

Of all lifestyle changes a pregnant woman should make, stopping drinking is perhaps the most important. Studies by the Department of

Health and Human Services show a direct relationship between the amount of alcohol consumed during a pregnancy and the potential of complications with a newborn child. This is especially evident when the woman drinks more than 1 alcoholic drink a day. The studies also show that a woman who drinks too much risks having a low-birth-weight baby or a child with congenital abnormalities such as mental retardation.

Since it's often difficult to tell how much is "too much," most pediatricians, family physicians, and obstetricians say that *any* alcohol consumed during a pregnancy has the potential to harm your unborn child. Mothers sometimes ask if an occasional glass of wine will hurt, and we have to say, "Probably not." But the key word here is *probably*. We can't be sure, so the advice has to be that expectant mothers *not* drink.

What are the effects of cigarette smoking during a pregnancy?

Like drinking, cigarette smoking has the potential to cause harm. Smoking during pregnancy increases the chance of having children with low birth weight and possible congenital abnormalities. It is certain that cigarette smoking harms the mother, and the inability to maintain an adequate oxygen flow because of the cigarette smoking points to potential harm to the unborn child.

So, it's obvious that the best advice for pregnant women is that habits such as drinking alcohol and smoking cigarettes should be stopped. Of course, some who drink moderately and smoke during pregnancy will have totally healthy children. But why risk it? If there is even the slightest chance that either of these habits can cause potential harm to the unborn child, they're best left alone.

FETAL DIAGNOSTIC TESTS

What is a sonogram?

A sonogram is a diagnostic test that can be used during certain phases of the pregnancy to examine the shape of the unborn child. Sound waves from a small instrument are bounced through the woman's uterus and then reflected back, creating a picture of the outline or shape of the child on a video monitor. A sonogram is painless and in most cases causes no harm to the child. Sonograms are used for various reasons, the most common being to detect whether the child is a male or female. Other diagnostic uses of the sonogram are the detection of twins, the detection of potential fetal abnormalities, and the determination of the unborn child's position in the uterus.

57

What is amniocentesis?

During the last decade, amniocentesis has revolutionized pregnancy for older women and for women at risk of having children with congenital disorders. In amniocentesis, a specimen of the amniotic fluid (the fluid surrounding the unborn child) is removed through a needle. This fluid, which contains all the genetic information about the child, is analyzed, and potential birth defects can be discovered. This procedure is performed early in the pregnancy, after the 16th week.

Women over 35 are especially interested in amniocentesis because of the possibility of recognizing potential for delivering a Down's syndrome baby. This is the major fetal abnormality that causes concern in older pregnant women.

Is there any risk to the child during amniocentesis? According to leading authorities, the risk of an abortion being created because of the procedure is very low.

CHILDBIRTH

What is a birthing center?

It is a special center specifically designed for the delivery of babies. At the center, trained nurses assist women who wish to deliver through natural childbirth. Many of these women would otherwise opt to deliver their babies at home. They are generally followed by an obstetrician or family physician throughout pregnancy, and near the time of delivery, are referred to the birthing center, where they are evaluated by the staff until time for delivery. During delivery, trained nurses or midwives closely observe, making sure no complications arise. If no problems occur, the woman delivers her child without anesthesia or drugs. Once the child is delivered, both mother and child return home to continue their care under the supervision of their own physician.

What is a birthing chair?

For centuries, women delivered their babies in a squatting position. This seemed to be the most comfortable for them and apparently did not cause any difficulties with the delivery. In fact, it is the most natural position a woman can assume, and some studies of other cultures show there is less discomfort and greater control of contractions. In order to duplicate this sitting position, a birthing chair has been introduced. In the chair, the woman sits upright at approximately a 45° angle while her legs are supported on either side with special stirrups. During labor, the bottom of the chair is comfortably flat, and when it is time for the child to be born, a special trapdoor is released to give greater access to the vagina for the delivery. When the birthing chair is used, the child is born downward rather than in the "modern" position where the woman is lying flat and the child is delivered straightforward. Under controlled circumstances, the birthing chair seems to give greater control and comfort during labor and delivery.

Who should deliver my baby?

The medical profession feels that a well-qualified physician should at least be in control of the delivery; that is, he or she should be available to supervise the delivery and handle any potential complications. But many women point out that physicians were not used for the delivery of babies until approximately 200 years ago and that it's certainly acceptable to have trained assistants rather than physicians. The medical profession's answer to this argument is that the physician is better trained to anticipate any problems involving labor, delivery, and immediate care of the newborn child.

Many women and nurse professionals believe that a well-qualified nurse or nurse midwife can certainly accomplish the same thing without the expense and inconvenience of being delivered by a physician. Nurse midwifery is on the upswing in this country, and with the growing interest in natural childbirth (often at home), nurse midwifery is certainly becoming an alternative.

I cannot say for sure which of these alternatives is best; however, we must agree on certain facts. Probably 95% of all deliveries are routine enough to be handled by almost anyone. We have all heard of healthy children being delivered by cab drivers and frantic husbands. I'm not worried about that 95%. What concerns me is the 5% of complicated deliveries that require medical expertise to ensure a healthy outcome. If we were able to anticipate which 5 out of 100 women would have complicated deliveries, then the other 95 could be delivered in just about any fashion they wished. The problem is that many times we *can't* anticipate complications during delivery. We can certainly make the blanket statement that any woman who is in a high-risk pregnancy or who has had problems with previous deliveries should be under the direct supervision of a physician.

The decision to utilize birthing centers, birthing chairs, or nurse midwives must ultimately be made by the woman. I strongly suggest she discuss this with the physician who has followed her during her pregnancy. As long as all the facts are known and a joint decision is made by mother and physician, a healthy outcome of the pregnancy and delivery should be assured.

59

How long will my labor be?

At approximately the 9th month of all pregnancies, the phenomenon of labor will begin, signaling the pending delivery of the child. Although many of the chemical and physiological changes that take place in the pregnancy are known, it is still somewhat of a mystery as to exactly why labor begins at the time it does.

As to how long your labor will be—no one can really tell, but there are some guidelines. If this is your 1st child, your vaginal canal is fairly tight and your cervix (the mouth of the womb) is fairly firm. Statistically, women who are delivering their 1st child will have longer labor than women who are delivering their 3rd or 4th child. Labor can last anywhere from 6 to 48 hours. Your physician will check you during your labor and examine the mouth of the womb to see how soft it is becoming and how much it is opening or dilating. The speed at which your cervix softens and dilates determines how long your labor will take.

Why do doctors monitor my baby during labor?

Fetal monitoring, a process by which the baby's heart rate and the strength of the contractions are simultaneously watched, was once utilized only for high-risk pregnancies. Today, fetal monitoring is fairly standard for all pregnancies because of the vast amount of information that can be gathered to ensure that all women, not just those at risk, will have a healthy labor and deliver a healthy child.

Physicians have been able to determine standards for strength of contractions and response of the fetal heart rate. When the strength of the contraction pattern is outside the norm or when the fetal heart rate response is abnormal, this could mean potential problems in the latter stages of labor. If these abnormalities are present, they alert the physician, who continues frequent monitoring on the outside chance that intervention in the labor will have to occur either by chemically inducing increased contractions or by performing a cesarean section.

Will the father be able to attend the birth?

Many years ago, fathers-to-be were almost never present at the delivery, although old movies showed them standing in the living room wringing their hands while a physician or a neighbor delivered the baby in the bedroom.

But with the resurgence of interest in natural deliveries (without the use of medications or delivery by forceps), men now are going into the delivery room. I have always felt the delivery of a child is a very special experience that should be shared by both mother and father. Seeing the child immediately upon delivery seems to facilitate a great deal of closeness and bonding between father and child, which is just as important as the bonding between mother and child.

More and more hospitals and physicians are openly encouraging fathers to attend deliveries. As you choose a doctor and a hospital, you might want to ask their policy on this subject. I feel that any father who wishes to attend a delivery should have that opportunity.

How can I know if I will need a cesarean section?

A cesarean section is an operation performed by a physician for the delivery of a child who cannot be delivered vaginally. The mother is given either general anesthesia or spinal anesthesia to numb her from the lower chest downward. The physician then makes an incision through the lower belly right over the uterus. The uterus is opened, the child and placenta are delivered, and the uterus and skin are sewn back up.

A cesarean section is used when there is pending danger to both mother and child and immediate delivery is indicated. Most often, this is for reasons of pelvic disproportion—when the woman's pelvis or birth canal is too small to deliver the child. A cesarean section is safe and acceptable; however, it should be used only under specific circumstances. The use of a cesarean section just to deliver a child on a "convenient" or preferred date and time is simply not good medical care.

Is it normal to be a little afraid before the delivery?

Yes. Most women, especially during their 1st pregnancy, are apprehensive before the delivery because they do not know what to expect. Many fear pain and discomfort. However, a great deal of a woman's fear as her pregnancy nears its end depends on the relationship she has with her physician and with her husband. A knowing, caring relationship, in which information has been shared with all 3 parties, tends to reduce the fear.

There is some discomfort associated with labor and delivery. For many it is significant but seems to be balanced for most women by the excitement and anticipation of giving birth. Men need to understand that this is sometimes a very painful and frightening time—a little understanding and caring go a long way.

Many woman ask if their pain can be eased with medication. The answer is yes. However, remember that any medication given during labor also goes through the umbilical cord to the unborn child. The physician must be careful not to oversedate or overmedicate to the point of slowing down the strength and frequency of the contractions or sedating the unborn child. This is where the relationship between the mother and physician is critical. The physician will try to make the labor and delivery as comfortable as possible for the mother, but certainly will not endanger the unborn child just to relieve the pain of the mother. It is a fine line that needs to be handled with expertise and care.

AGE AND PREGNANCY

How old is too old to get pregnant?

Many years ago, physicians counseled women to complete their families before they were in their early to mid-30's. The major reason behind this was that the older a woman is, the greater her chance of delivering a child with congenital abnormalities, especially Down's syndrome. According to Dr. Owen Rennert of Oklahoma College of Medicine, a 35-year-old woman having her 1st child runs around a 2% chance of having a child with a serious birth defect—twice that of a 25 year old. Women over 40 have a 1 in 100 chance of delivering a Down's syndrome infant compared to 1 in 885 at age 30. The frequency of Down's syndrome increases with the age of the mother; these percentages take a dramatic leap when women are over 35 and especially over 40.

However, with the increased use of birth control and the decision to delay getting pregnant because of career plans, many women between the ages of 32 and 35 are having their 1st child. This is becoming increasingly common and acceptable both socially and medically. During the last 10 years, the number of women waiting until after 30 to become mothers has almost doubled. In fact, many in their late 30's and even in their early 40's get pregnant and deliver normal healthy children. Those women should understand the increased risk of delivering a Down's syndrome child; but as long as they are under the close supervision of a physician and understand the risk, they should, within reason, be able to elect when to begin a family.

Why do older women have a greater risk of delivering a child with birth defects?

Although most women over 35 will have healthy children, the reason for the greater risk is simple biology. A woman is born with ovaries that contain a preset number of egg cells called oocytes. Certain of these ripen into eggs and are available for fertilization with each menstrual cycle. The older a woman becomes, the older these oocytes become. Age, therefore, increases the chance that the "aged" eggs will not function properly when fertilized, thus causing a miscarriage or a birth defect.

BIRTH DEFECTS

What are some of the causes for a child being born with a birth defect?

The fear of having a child with a birth defect probably crosses the mind of almost anyone considering or entering parenthood. The incidence of birth defects today is about the same as it was 10 years ago. However, the public is much more knowledgeable about them, and the technology to manage many of these birth defects has advanced rapidly. Today babies with problems such as low birth weight, cystic fibrosis, and spina bifida are much more likely to live.

Only about 30% of birth defects can be traced to a specific cause. The remaining 70% are unknown. Of the 30% where the cause is known, approximately 20% are caused by a defect in the genes, 5% are attributable to chromosomal abnormalities, 1% to therapeutic irradiation, 2% to 3% to maternal conditions, and another 2% to 3% to drugs or environmental chemicals.

Of course, there is always a possibility that a child will be born with birth defects, but the overall chances and percentages favor a totally healthy baby. Frequent prenatal visits, the avoidance of unnecessary medications, and the avoidance of alcohol and drugs during pregnancy substantially increase the chances that you will have a healthy child.

What are the most common birth defects?

The most common congenital malformations seen today are cleft palate, clubfoot, and dislocated hip. Some degree of malformations are observed in 2% to 3% of all births, while chromosomal disorders (disorders related to abnormal genetic materials) are observed in approximately 1 of every 200 births. The most common chromosomal abnormality is Down's syndrome, which occurs in approximately 1 of every 1000 births.

If my child is born normal, does that mean he or she does not have any birth defects?

By and large the vast majority of birth defects are recognizable at birth. There are, however, a small percentage of congenital conditions that are not recognized until later in life. Many orthopedic problems, problems with the skeleton and joints, may not appear until later in the child's growth and development. But remember, if most of these are found early enough, corrective measures can be taken.

I have heard about children being born with heart defects. What are some of the most common heart malformations that occur at birth?

Congenital heart defects are present in some degree in about 1% of all births. The 2 most frequently diagnosed heart defects in newborn children are patent ductus arteriosus and ventricular septal defect.

To understand what a patent ductus arteriosus is, we must look at the unusual circulatory system of the child while it is still in the mother's uterus. Even though the heart is present, the blood flow through the unborn child's body is diverted from the lungs and goes directly from the heart to the major circulation system. This is because the unborn child's oxygen supply comes directly from the mother since its own lungs are not yet functioning. The connection between the heart and the general circulation that bypasses the lungs is called the ductus arteriosus. In most cases, as soon as the child takes its first breath, this little channel begins to close off and is generally completely closed within the first few days of life, but in some children this canal stays open and causes a heart murmur called a patent ductus arteriosus. This defect occurs in 12% of babies born with congenital heart defects and is twice as common in females as in males.

Returning again to the circulation of the unborn child, we know that the lower part of the heart is divided into two ventricles. Between the ventricles is a membrane wall called a septum. If this septum does not develop completely, it leaves a small hole between the ventricles, which is called a septal defect. If this opening does not close off after birth, it also causes a heart murmur. This heart murmur (ventricular septal defect) causes no problems in the vast majority of cases, but it can be significant enough to require surgery later in the child's life. It is found in 25% of all children with congenital heart defects.

There are, of course, more serious heart defects, but these are much less frequent. Remember, with modern medical and surgical technology, amazing results are being achieved.

3.

Taking Care of a Sick Child

FEVER

What causes fever in children?

Any elevation in the core temperature of the body is a fever. The primary cause of fever is the body's response to some form of infection. Both bacterial and viral infections can cause an elevation in temperature because of the materials, called toxins, they release. This elevation of the body's temperature can be noted through the use of a thermometer.

The normal temperature of the body is 98.6° Fahrenheit by an oral thermometer or 1° higher (100°) with a rectal thermometer. Of course, this can vary slightly from person to person; some children can have a temperature of 98.2° or 98.8° and still be considered normal.

But when there is infection, the temperature will generally rise. How much it rises depends upon the type of infection, but how high a temperature goes is generally not an indication of how sick the child is. Many viral illnesses that last only 2 to 3 days can cause an elevation of temperature up to 103° or 104°. The child is not seriously ill even though the temperature has risen that high. Other infections can cause a child to be very sick but may cause a rise in temperature to only 101° or 102°.

What is the best way to take my child's temperature?

Depending upon the age of the child, a temperature can be taken either in the rectum, under the arm, or in the mouth. Rectal temperatures are normally taken of infants too small to hold the thermometer in their mouths. As the child gets a little older, taking the

65

temperature under the arm is acceptable. When the child reaches the age of 3 or 4 years, taking the temperature by mouth is the most accurate. A thermometer with a more rounded end bulb should be used for rectal temperature checks as the danger of tearing the rectum is reduced.

All parents should remember that rectal temperatures are a little higher than temperatures taken by mouth. A rectal temperature of 100° Fahrenheit may be totally normal in an infant. The axillary temperature (under the arm) is usually 1° lower than the temperature taken by mouth.

If you are taking the rectal temperature of your child, remember to coat the bulb of the thermometer with petroleum jelly. Gently insert the thermometer no more than 1″. Hold the thermometer in place for approximately 2 to 3 minutes before removing.

If you are taking the temperature under the arm, place the bulb of the thermometer under the upper armpit of the child and hold the thermometer snugly in place by placing the arm close to the body. The armpit should be dry at the time of taking the temperature. Generally you should wait 3 to 4 minutes before removing.

If you are taking your child's temperature by mouth, place the bulb end of the oral thermometer under the tongue. Tell the child to close the mouth but not to bite on the thermometer. Leave in place for approximately 2 to 3 minutes.

Is a fever harmful to my child?

Fever is nature's way of telling us that there is some infection, either viral or bacterial, going on within the body. Remember, fever is a symptom of a disease just like coughing, diarrhea, and vomiting. Fever doesn't harm a child unless it gets out of control; an elevated temperature doesn't necessarily mean that the child is critically ill.

If your child develops a fever, do not panic. Simply look at the child and determine whether or not there are any associated symptoms such as a cough, an earache, a sore throat, difficulty in breathing, or a change in behavior. Then begin treatment of the fever. If the temperature does not return to normal after 24 hours or if unassociated symptoms persist, notify your physician.

What is the best way to treat fever in my child?

Aspirin and acetaminophen are the 2 basic medications used to treat fever.

Acetylsalicylic acid (aspirin) is a widely prescribed drug for lowering a child's temperature and can be given in liquid, suppository, or tablet form. The amount of aspirin used to treat a child's fever depends on the child's age and weight. Aspirin bottles generally state the appropriate dose, but a basic guideline is that any child 1 year of age can be treated with 1 grain of aspirin, which is equal to 1 baby aspirin. For every year of age, an additional baby aspirin can be given. For example, a 3-year-old child could be given 3 baby aspirin approximately every 4 hours to lower temperature. Children under a year old can be given aspirin in either liquid or suppository form. It is generally recommended that aspirin not be given more often than every 4 hours. A good guideline to use is to give the aspirin until the child's fever has remained normal for 24 hours.

Acetaminophen is also found in tablet, liquid, or suppository form and it is rapidly becoming the most widely prescribed medication to treat a child's fever. The dosage for acetaminophen follows the basic guidelines used for aspirin—your child's age and weight. Below you will find basic guidelines for both medications, but I strongly recommend that you review the directions on the bottle before using either and talk with your pediatrician or family physician.

When should I treat a fever in my child?

The main reason to treat fever of less than 103° is to make the child more comfortable. Fever over 103° needs to be treated to keep it from rising any higher.

Many parents believe that any time the child's temperature rises above 98.6° they should immediately begin aspirin or acetaminophen. This helps the child feel better, but treating the fever is not mandatory to make the illness go away. The fever will dissipate when the infection has run its course.

What if my child's fever does not respond to either aspirin or acetaminophen?

Many times the child's fever will not go down, even with giving aspirin or acetaminophen every 4 hours. If this happens, you may want to try what I call the alternating treatment for fever. Give the proper dose (according to child's age and weight) of aspirin, and after 2 hours, give a similar dose of acetaminophen. Alternate doses of aspirin and acetaminophen every 2 hours until the child's fever begins to respond.

Another way to treat an unresponsive fever is to place the child in a tepid bath, it will cool the child's skin or surface temperature and allow the fever to dissipate through the skin.

Alcohol sponge baths can also be used on the same principle: the alcohol is sponged on the surface of the skin, evaporates from the heat of the body, and causes a lowering of the core temperature. Be cautious not to get the alcohol in your child's eyes.

If your child's temperature does not respond even to the alternating therapy after 48 hours, consult your physician.

Are there any times that I should not use aspirin?

Yes. Aspirin should never be given to a child who is suspected of having either "true flu" (flu carried by specific influenza viruses), or chicken pox. The reason for not using salicylates in these 2 particular illnesses has to do with the development of Reye's syndrome. Reye's syndrome is an acute condition characterized by sudden vomiting, violent headaches, and unusual behavior in children who appear to be recovering from just a mild viral illness. Reye's syndrome is a rare disease, but when it occurs, it is considered life-threatening.

There has been a close association between the use of aspirin in children with chicken pox or true influenza and the development of Reye's syndrome. Both the American Academy of Pediatrics and the American Academy of Family Physicians strongly recommend that aspirin not be given to children with chicken pox or influenza because of the potential of developing Reye's syndrome.

Does that mean that aspirin can cause Reye's syndrome?

Medical experts have concluded that aspirin does not *cause* Reye's syndrome, but aspirin has been associated with its development. Extensive studies have been undertaken to try to find the causes of the syndrome, but the only thing that seems to be similar in all cases of Reye's syndrome is that they have followed illnesses such as chicken pox and influenza and occur more frequently in children who have been given aspirin during these 2 illnesses. The association cannot be ignored, so physicians strongly recommend the use of acetaminophen to treat fever with true influenza and chicken pox.

Why not avoid aspirin in all cases of treating fever in children?

Many parents have applied the warning about Reye's syndrome to all illnesses and they never give aspirin to their children. However, there are no contrary indications to using aspirin to treat the fever of anything except true influenza and chicken pox. In fact, aspirin is often a more acceptable medication than acetaminophen. Aspirin is the drug of choice in treating children with rheumatic fever and rheumatoid arthritis, and it is also much better than acetaminophen for treating the general aches and pains associated with many illnesses.

The best way to determine whether or not to give your child aspirin is to consult your physician. If there is reason to think that your child may have chicken pox or true influenza, always consult your physician before giving aspirin.

What are febrile convulsions?

Febrile convulsions, or seizures, are related to the rapid onset of fever in some children. We are not exactly sure why certain children are more susceptible to those convulsions, but their occurrence can be very frightening to parents. A child may appear to be well, then develop a fever, and within several hours have a fit or seizure. This is generally a shaking type of convulsion that lasts several seconds to several minutes. After the convulsion is over, the child is somewhat sleepy and drowsy but otherwise okay.

Febrile convulsions are seen most often in children between the ages of 18 months and 4 years. Approximately 10% to 15% of all children will at some time have a febrile seizure. These seizures are very frightening to the child and the parents, but they in no way indicate that the child will always have problems with seizures or will develop epilepsy. Also, when a child has a seizure, it does not mean that the infection is any worse.

If your child has a febrile seizure, report it to your physician who will generally give the child a thorough examination, including a neurological evaluation. If the preliminary examination is normal, the physician will keep an eye on the child and show the parents how to cope.

Some children will have repeated seizures that require special treatment. If a child has a 2nd febrile seizure, the physician may recommend the use of a medication called phenobarbital at the 1st sign of a fever in the child. The phenobarbital, a sedative, is used not to treat the fever but to prevent the possibility of a repeated seizure. If a child has more than 2 or 3 seizures, the physician will probably want to perform certain tests to make sure there are no underlying signs of epilepsy. The vast majority of children with febrile seizures have absolutely *no* indication of underlying epilepsy nor will they develop epilepsy in the future. Febrile seizures are frightening, but they are not dangerous.

INFECTIONS

What is an upper respiratory infection?

Upper respiratory infections, or colds, are the most common illnesses your child will have. The number of colds a child will have depends upon age and exposure to other children. A 6 month old who is cared for in a nursery with other children will usually have more colds than a child who is not. Most children have between 5 and 10 colds a year until they are approximately 10 years of age.

Colds are caused by viruses, and to date, there is no effective immunization or single medication that prevents or cures them. Penicillin and other antibiotics are not beneficial in the treatment of upper respiratory infections unless a complication such as an ear or lung infection exists.

Colds generally begin with some nasal congestion and a runny nose. Other symptoms are red and runny eyes (conjunctivitis), sore throat, sneezing, and coughing (especially at night).

You should notify your doctor when your child has a cold *if* he or she seems very weak and sick, has labored breathing without a congested nose, cries and moans as if in pain for several hours, or complains of ear pain.

How do I treat my child's cold?

The treatment of a common cold is entirely symptomatic and is undertaken to make your child feel more comfortable. If your child's cold is very mild and there is no discomfort, little or no treatment may be necessary. Remember, you can't cure a cold—you can only keep the child as comfortable as possible until it runs its course.

Perhaps the most troublesome symptoms of a cold are nasal congestion and a cough. If these become bothersome, use oral or nasal decongestants prescribed by your physician. For an infant's stuffy nose, the best treatment is the use of saline nose drops. These drops can be used in association with a nasal syringe to clear the child's nostrils of secretions. You can make saline nose drops by simply placing ½ teaspoon salt in ½ pint water. Boil this solution, let it cool, and place it in the refrigerator. Use a nose dropper to place 1 to 2 drops of the solution in each nostril before using the nasal syringe. In children over 6–7 years, nasal congestion can also be treated with the use of oral decongestant/antihistamine medications. For these children, medications can be purchased over the counter and, if used properly, can help your child feel better. Do not use these medications for more then 2 or 3 days, though.

The rattling cough associated with many colds is caused by nasal secretions dripping down the back of the throat and into the chest. The use of antihistamines that stop the nasal congestion will often relieve the rattling cough. If it does not, try a combination decongestant/cough medicine. If your child's cough persists, especially if it is associated with a fever, consult your physician.

Why do so many children have frequent ear infections?

The anatomy of a child's ears is entirely different from that of an adult. We all have a small tube, called the eustachian tube, that runs from the middle ear to the back of the throat. The purpose of this tube is to equalize the pressure behind the eardrum with the outer environment. All of us have experienced the functioning of the eustachian tube when we go up in an elevator or in an airplane and our ears pop. This popping sensation is caused by the opening and closing of the eustachian tube.

In young children, especially infants, the eustachian tube is very short and wide open, creating access for any viral or bacterial agents in the back of the throat or the nose to get into the eustachian tube and seep into the middle ear. The eustachian tube is also highly susceptible to closing up very rapidly, and once it closes up, pressure builds in the middle ear. The combination of the pressure and the possibility of bacteria seeping up through the tube set up a perfect environment for the development of middle ear infections in children.

How can I tell if my child has developed a middle ear infection?

Most children with middle ear infections will complain of ear pain. Older children will tell you that their ears hurt, but younger children, especially infants, may be unusually restless or tug at 1 or both ears. The vast majority of middle ear infections occur after the child has developed a runny nose or coldlike symptoms. Most middle ear infections are accompanied by fever. So, a child who has recently developed a cold, complains of ear pain or tugs at the ears, and has a persistent fever may have developed a middle ear infection.

If your child complains of ear pain and you are not sure whether or not it is from the middle ear, here is a simple test: gently tug on the child's earlobe. If the pain gets worse, the ear pain is probably coming from an external infection and not from the middle ear. If tugging on the ear does not make the pain worse and the child has the other symptoms mentioned, the child has probably developed a middle ear infection.

How are middle ear infections treated?

Middle ear infections in children must be treated with antibiotics because the fluid behind the middle ear has become infected. The type of antibiotic your physician uses will depend upon the age of the child. In children under 5 years of age, the infection is most often caused by the bacteria *Hemophilus influenzae,* and most physicians will use either ampicillin or a sulfa medication.

71

In children 6 to 8 years of age, the most common bacteria is pneumococcus. For children this age and older, your physician may elect to use either penicillin or erythromycin.

The use of antihistamines and decongestants in middle ear infections is somewhat controversial. Some physicians believe that when antihistamines are used in association with the antibiotic the child's ear infections seem to clear better. However, research indicates that the primary medication needed to clear the infection is the antibiotic; the antihistamine does not seem to facilitate the recovery.

Why is it so important to treat middle ear infections?

Every time an infection occurs, infected fluid builds up in the middle ear. If this infection is not treated effectively and rapidly, the fluid in the middle ear can begin to congeal or thicken. The hearing mechanism is carried out by 3 small bones in the middle ear that vibrate when sound hits the eardrum. If fluid surrounds these small bones because of congestion or infection, the bones do not move as freely, and the child will not hear as well out of that ear. If repeated infections occur, the fluid can become thick and gluelike, and it can be very difficult to remove.

For this reason, it is extremely important to treat these infections promptly and properly and to follow up to make sure that all the fluid has left and that the eardrum is functioning normally.

Why do some children have to have tubes placed in their ears?

Sometimes the fluid in the middle ear gets so thick that it simply can't be removed with medications that open up the eustachian tube. When this occurs, physicians sometimes have to drain the fluid out of the ears by placing tubes in them.

Myringotomy is performed by making a small nick or cut in the eardrum. Then a small plastic tube is slid through the cut, giving an open canal from the middle ear to the outside. This small tube, which will replace the functioning of the eustachian tube until the middle ear drains, is generally left in place for 6 months to 1 year. Many times these tubes will begin to gradually work their way out of the eardrum themselves and can fall out or be removed by the physician. The placement of these tubes in no way interferes with the child's ability to hear and may keep the child from having permanent hearing problems.

The placement of these tubes should be handled by experienced physicians such as ENT (ear, nose, and throat) specialists. Used properly, the tubes can potentially save the child's hearing.

What is swimmer's ear?

Swimmer's ear is an infection of the outer ear canal, the passageway leading from the outer ear down to the eardrum. Swimmer's ear can be caused by bacterial or fungal infections and is contracted when children swim a lot, especially in lakes or unchlorinated pools. However, it can be caused by water that gets into the ear after a bath or shower.

An easy way to determine if your child has swimmer's ear is to perform this simple test: tug very gently on the earlobe. If that increases the pain, you're probably dealing with swimmer's ear. The reason the pain gets worse is that tugging on the ear also tugs on the ear canal and irritates the infected area.

Swimmer's ear is treated with drops, not oral antibiotics. The ear drops reduce the irritation and treat the suspected fungal or bacterial infection. Placing 1 to 2 drops in each ear, 4 times a day for approximately 5 to 7 days, is highly effective in reducing both the pain and the infection. Of course, there should be no swimming until the infection clears.

For children who have repeated episodes of swimmer's ear, certain medications can be used to reduce the occurrences of ear infections after swimming. These medications help dry the ear after swimming, eliminating the nice, moist place for bacteria or fungus to grow. Consult your physician for ear drops to be used during the swimming season.

ALLERGIES

How can I tell if my child has allergies?

The symptoms of allergies and colds are quite similar—runny nose, itchy/watery eyes, sneezing, and sometimes a dry, hacking cough. Perhaps the best way to tell whether or not these symptoms are caused by allergies is to determine when the "cold" occurs. If your child has "colds" primarily in the spring and early fall, the symptoms could be caused by an environmental allergy. If your child has these same symptoms that last periodically throughout the year, then it is more probable that these are just the normal colds that your child will have from time to time.

If you are concerned that your child might have allergies, consult your physician. Your pediatrician or family physician can run some basic tests to at least suggest whether or not your child's symptoms could be caused by allergies.

If your child has frequent chest infections, asthmatic attacks, or ear infections, your physician may recommend that a thorough evaluation be undertaken by an allergy specialist. At this time, the specialist can perform tests to determine if there is any specific thing your child is allergic to. If there is, then allergy shots might be needed to desensitize, or lessen, your child's response to those particular environmental factors. When the child is desensitized, the occurrence of complications such as bronchitis, asthma, or ear infections is less frequent so that your child's overall health improves.

SORE THROAT

What causes sore throats?

Sore throats are fairly common among children because they can be associated with the common cold, viral infections, or bacterial infections. The symptoms of sore throats do not help very much in determining which of these is the cause. The pain and fever accompanying a sore throat from a viral infection do not differ significantly from the pain and fever accompanying a sore throat from a bacterial infection. Strep throat is caused by streptococcal bacteria, and a common way to diagnose it is to discover the presence of a coating on the tonsils. However, many viral infections are associated with white patches, or exudate, on the tonsils. The only absolute way a physician can determine whether or not a child has strep throat is to take a throat culture. A sterile swab is used to obtain some of the exudate from the tonsils, and then this exudate is placed in a special type of culture medium that will allow the streptococcal bacteria to grow if it is present. (Throat cultures take about 24 hours to give us the answer. Recently, a newer method of culturing throats has been developed that takes less than 30 minutes.)

Another, less accurate, way to diagnose strep throat is to take a blood test. A bacterial infection such as strep throat sometimes causes the white blood cell count to rise above normal. (A viral infection such as the common cold or influenza most often causes the white blood cell count to be lower than normal.) But even though taking a white blood cell count is quicker than taking a throat culture, it is not as accurate in determining whether or not streptococcal infections are present.

Because streptococcal infections are bacterial, they are treated with antibiotics, usually penicillin or erythromycin. Once antibiotics are begun, the infection will begin to clear in 1 or 2 days. However, to prevent a relapse, the antibiotics *must* be taken for 7 to 10 full days.

If the sore throat is caused by a virus, it will generally get better in 2 to 3 days with aspirin or acetaminophen and cold fluids to soothe the throat. If the child is old enough, gargling can help.

COUGHS

What should I do when my child develops a cough?

There are basically 2 types of coughs in children, and the treatment depends upon the cause.

The 1st type is the nonproductive cough. This is generally associated with most upper respiratory infections and is characterized by a dry hacking. The nonproductive cough gets worse at night because the child lies down and all that congestion in the head drips to the back of the throat, irritating the cough mechanism. During the day, the child may cough a few times but not nearly as much as at night. The best way to treat this type of cough is to stop the postnasal drainage. Giving the child antihistamines at bedtime to dry up the nasal secretions will often prevent the cough, and a humidifier at the bedside can also help.

The 2nd type is the productive cough. This more significant and potentially harmful cough is associated with rattling in the chest, the production of phlegm, and sometimes difficulty in breathing. A productive cough generally means that the infection has gotten down into the chest and may indicate an infection of the bronchial tubes (bronchitis) or an infection of the lung tissue itself (pneumonia). The productive cough generally needs to be treated with a cough expectorant to help rid the lungs of the congestion. Never give a child with a productive cough a lot of antihistamines because they dry up the congestion in the chest and make it more difficult for the child to get rid of the infection.

Consult your physician when your child has a persistent cough that is unresponsive to simple measures; when the cough is associated with fever for more than 2 days; when your child has difficulty breathing; or when a whistling or wheezing sound develops in the child's breathing.

MONONUCLEOSIS

What is mononucleosis?

Mononucleosis, often referred to as "the kissing disease," is a specific viral disease thought to be caused by the Epstein-Barr virus. Early symptoms of mononucleosis are often similar to those of strep throat or a bad cold. Sometimes the fever will rise to 102° or 103°, and the throat will have a very thick coating or exudate on it.

A classic symptom of mononucleosis is a generalized swelling of the lymph nodes in the neck, under the arms, and in the groin. Another symptom is tremendous fatigue or a listless feeling. Mononucleosis generally affects young people in their early to late teens.

Because mononucleosis is caused by a virus, there is no cure for the illness, but it can be helped by bed rest and proper diet. Years ago,

75

young people with "mono" would be put to bed for 2 to 3 months for recuperation, but we now realize that this is not necessary as long as they take care of themselves during the early stages.

There are, however, some complications of mononucleosis that can cause problems. Hepatitis (inflammation of the liver) and an enlargement of the spleen can complicate the course of mononucleosis. Your physician will want to make sure that neither complication occurs.

DIAPER RASH

What can I do about my child's diaper rash?

There are many causes of diaper rash, but the most common are (1) the excessive ammonia that is formed on the wet diaper and the skin by a bacterial reaction with the urine; (2) fungal infections such as the common yeast infection; (3) allergies, specifically allergies to the materials in the diaper; and (4) bacterial infections that are associated with pustules or yellowish bumps.

Many remedies are offered for the treatment of diaper rashes, but it is generally useful to remember that the less applied to the baby's skin, the better. In primitive societies where diapers are not worn, diaper rash is almost nonexistent.

A lot of parents will wonder whether or not the child's diet is related to the formation of diaper rashes. As far as I know, there is no evidence that a child's diet either causes or prevents it.

Mildly irritated rashes in the diaper area are common in almost all children and generallly require no treatment. However, if the condition persists, you can follow the directions listed below. A standard ointment such as zinc oxide or A and D ointment can be used for the treatment of mild forms and can be effective in the prevention of some of the irritative diaper rashes. A mild petroleum jelly can also be applied in a very thin coating to protect the child's bottom and genital region from urine irritation.

Special prescription medications are needed for diaper rashes caused by fungus and bacteria. Your physician should be contacted if a diaper rash fails to respond to the zinc oxide or A and D ointment or if it begins to look worse.

To prevent the chances of your child's having diaper rash use the following guidelines:
• Change your baby's diaper as soon as he or she wets or soils it, or at least every 3 hours during the day. You should check the diaper at night, too, before you go to sleep. If it's wet or soiled, change it.

- At each diaper change, cleanse the area gently and thoroughly using soap and water and then pat the skin dry. Avoid using soaps that contain perfumes and other additives. They are harsh to an infant's skin, and your child could be allergic to them.
- When your child is in the crib, bed, or playpen, avoid using plastic pants. If you are using disposable diapers, remove the plastic cover. Fasten the diaper loosely to allow the moisture next to the skin to evaporate. During the day, the child could be left in the playpen without diapers.
- Talcum powder or corn starch can be gently applied to the skin in the diaper area to increase the absorption of moisture. If you use talcum powder, take care when applying it so that the baby does not inhale the powder particles and irritate the lungs.

Are cloth or disposable diapers better?

Doctors agree that for the most part the only children who never have diaper rash are those who never wear diapers. Children kept in cloth diapers seem to be as likely to develop diaper rashes as those kept in disposable diapers. Of course, some children are allergic to the materials in disposable diapers. This can be identified by a persistent diaper rash that fails to respond to any of the normal treatments.

On the other hand, some children may be allergic to cloth diapers or, more exactly, to the materials that the cloth diapers are washed in. Using strong detergents to wash cloth diapers can increase the possibility of your child's developing an irritative diaper rash. If you use cloth diapers, wash the diapers at home using a mild detergent such as Ivory Snow and an extra hot-water rinse. Avoid harsh detergents, presoaks, bleaches, or fabric softeners since they may leave residue in the diaper that can irritate your child's skin.

The advantage of cloth diapers is that they can be worn without plastic pants. But the plastic cover can be removed from most disposable diapers, too.

DIARRHEA AND VOMITING

How can I determine if my child is having diarrhea?

The term *diarrhea* is often misunderstood. *Diarrhea* means that the "stools are more loose, more watery, and more frequent than normal." But determining how this very simple definition fits your child can be complicated. The key is recognizing what is normal for your baby. If there is a change from your child's normal pattern to a more frequent or more watery bowel movement, then it is diarrhea.

The most common misconception is that if a baby has more than 4 or 5 bowel movements a day the child must be sick with diarrhea. This is nonsense. Many infants will have bowel movements after each feeding, which can account for 4, 5, or up to 8 bowel movements a day. Other children will have bowel movements every 2 to 3 days and be perfectly comfortable and normal. In the 1st instance, the child would have to have 10 or 12 bowel movements a day before the definition of diarrhea would fit. If the child in the 2nd case had 2 to 3 bowel movements every day, that child would probably have diarrhea.

Breast-fed babies usually have softer, less firm stools than bottle-fed babies. Both breast- and bottle-fed infants have softer, less firm stools than older children and adults.

So the trick in determining whether or not your child has diarrhea is determining whether or not there has been a change in your child's normal stool pattern. If there is no change, then your child's pattern may be perfectly normal.

What are the main causes of infant diarrhea?

There are several causes of infant diarrhea. Determining the specific cause has a good deal to do with the recommendation for the treatment at home. For instance, teething can cause a change in a child's normal bowel pattern. Many children will have mild diarrhea with every new tooth formed. In fact, some parents can actually predict when a child is about to cut a new tooth because of the change in the normal bowel pattern.

Overfeeding is probably the most common cause of mild diarrhea. Overfeeding can lead to increased vomiting and to an increase in the frequency of stools.

Another common cause of infant diarrhea is the use of antibiotics to treat certain infections, such as when an ear infection is treated with the antibiotic ampicillin. Ampicillin can cause a mild case of diarrhea in the child because of its effect on the normal bacteria within the child's intestinal tract. Don't be overly concerned if a mild case of diarrhea develops when your child is placed on antibiotics for an ear infection.

Diarrhea can also be associated with some of the more frequent infections your child may contract, such as with an upper respiratory infection, a sore throat, or an ear infection.

Perhaps the most serious type of diarrhea is that associated with gastroenteritis, an infection caused by a virus in the digestive tract. With this illness, your child will run a mild fever, perhaps have some vomiting, and have diarrhea characterized by increased frequency and looseness of stools and occasional complaints of cramping.

When should I use medications to treat my child's diarrhea?

For children over 6 or 7 years of age, the use of some of the over-the-counter antidiarrheal agents can be highly effective in decreasing the cramping and slowing down the diarrhea. However, these medications should never be used in children under 2 years of age unless you consult your physician.

Medications for adults who develop diarrhea are generally too strong for children. Again, these medications should never be used in young children without consulting your physician.

You can give doses of over-the-counter antidiarrheal medications to an older child as long as you follow the directions on the label according to the child's weight and age. And, of course, if the diarrhea does not respond to treatment, call your physician.

Why is it so important to recognize and treat diarrhea?

The main reason that we want to make sure to recognize true diarrhea and institute treatment is to prevent dehydration (the excessive loss of fluids in the body).

In our bodies, there is a very delicate balance between the amount of fluids and electrolytes such as sodium and potassium. If this delicate balance is interrupted through the excessive loss of fluids from either diarrhea or vomiting, the child can experience some significant symptoms.

Here are some of the more common symptoms of dehydration in a child:

- A change in behavior such as an increase in listlessness, sleepiness, or irritability
- A decrease in the amount of urine produced each day
- A persistent fever, unresponsive to normal medications
- Very dry lips and tongue and a decrease in the amount of saliva
- Poor sucking reflex
- Increased rate and shallowness of respirations

If your child is experiencing diarrhea and vomiting, the chances of dehydration are increased. If your child shows any of these symptoms, you must notify your physician immediately.

What can I do to treat diarrhea or vomiting and prevent dehydration?

The best way to prevent dehydration is to recognize its potential occurrence. Any time your child is suffering from severe diarrhea, especially when combined with vomiting, the potential for dehydration is there.

If your child develops true diarrhea, he or she should be taken off all solid foods, milk, and milk products and put on a diet of clear liquids. Clear liquids are any liquids that you can hold up to the light and see through, such as ginger ale, tea, and Gatorade. Gatorade is especially good because it contains the vital electrolytes that your child loses with diarrhea and vomiting.

If you use cola or ginger ale, take the carbonation out because it can increase the chances of your child's vomiting. This can be done by shaking the cola, letting all the "fizz" out, and letting the open bottle sit for an hour.

As soon as your child develops diarrhea, place him or her on clear liquids immediately. As long as the child takes the clear liquids and does not start vomiting, the chances of dehydration are very slim. If, however, vomiting does occur and you notice a significant decrease in the amount of urine or an increase of other dehydration symptoms, notify your physician.

A special note: For young babies who develop rather severe cases of diarrhea a product called Pedialyte contains fluids as well as critical electrolytes. Small bottles of Pedialyte can be used to increase the amount of fluids and electrolytes your sick child is taking in and thus prevent dehydration.

What are some of the more common causes of vomiting in children?

Vomiting is a frequent symptom of gastroenteritis. Vomiting is also a common symptom of other infections such as strep throat, ear infections, or colds that produce a great deal of phlegm in the back of the throat.

If your child begins vomiting, the 1st thing to do is to stop giving the child anything by mouth. A child 5 years or older should probably go at least 1 to 2 hours without anything in the stomach before clear liquids are begun. Younger children can probably go an hour before you should try to institute the feedings of clear liquids. Many children who develop vomiting with gastrointestinal or other infections respond quite rapidly to simply taking them off solid foods, milk, and milk products and beginning clear liquids.

However, if your child continues to vomit despite the institution of clear liquids, or if the vomiting persists for more than 24 hours (especially in children under 5 years of age), consult your physician for the possibility of needing medications to treat the vomiting. These medications can be given in the form of suppositories and are highly effective.

Always consult your physician if vomiting persists, if it is associated with fever, or if it is associated with the symptoms of dehydration.

ACCIDENTAL POISONING

How can I prevent accidental poisonings?

According to the National Poison Control Center, each year in the United States there are at least 1 million cases of children ingesting toxic agents with the resulting loss of thousands of lives. In 1972, over 8000 children under the age of 5 required medical attention after ingesting poisonous amounts of aspirin. By 1982 this figure had dropped to 1700—a 78% decrease. Much of this drop can be attributed to the Poison Prevention Act that required child-resistant caps on all medications and many household products.

All parents should be aware of the importance of preventing accidental poisonings. Here are some suggested guidelines to prevent your child from becoming an accidental poisoning statistic:

- Be sure that all medications in your house (even a "common" medication such as aspirin) are placed under lock and key in a medicine cabinet. Store all cleaning preparations in a safe place. Consider placing them in a locked cabinet, too.
- Never refer to medication as candy. This may encourage your child to get some more "candy" when you are not around.
- If you have a toddler in the house, keep in mind the tot's ability (and inclination) to climb. Make sure that medications are under lock and key, not just kept on a high shelf.
- Never administer medication to your child in the dark without making sure that you are taking the medication from the proper bottle and giving the proper dosage.
- Check and double-check the calculated dose of medication to give your child.
- Have the phone number of your local poison control center, emergency room, and physician readily available by the phone.

How do you treat accidental poisonings?

Suppose that your child has gotten into some medication or a household substance that could potentially harm the child. What should you do? Every household that has children under the age of 10 should have

81

the number of the local poison control center listed next to each telephone *and* in another area of the house, such as inside the locked medicine cabinet. If you suspect that your child has taken some medication or accidently swallowed other potentially poisonous agents, immediately try to determine what and how much has been ingested and then call the poison control center. If a poison control center is not readily identifiable in your area, call your physician or local emergency room. Either the poison control center or your physician can give you recommended emergency treatments.

All families with children should have an adequate supply of ipecac on hand. Ipecac is a syrup that will induce vomiting. The proper dose of ipecac for your child can be easily calculated by following the directions on the bottle. There is a *warning,* however. Vomiting should *never* be induced in a child who has ingested a caustic material such as kerosene, gasoline, turpentine, paint thinner, or lye, because if the child vomits and then breathes some of the material into the lungs (aspirates), the lungs can be permanently damaged. If there is any question as to whether or not you should induce vomiting, consult the poison control center or your physician.

4.

Childhood Diseases and Immunizations

WHAT IS AN IMMUNIZATION?

The body has a variety of systems that perform a marvelous job of defending against certain illnesses. But for some diseases, the body's defense mechanism needs additional help.

An immunization is a safe, effective method of protecting against certain diseases. With this procedure, a very small portion of the agent that causes the disease is either injected into the body or taken orally. This stimulates the production of substances called antibodies that are used to fight off the infection. These antibodies become the body's defense mechanism against future exposure to the disease.

The protection that these antibodies produce is called immunity. After receiving the proper immunization, a child is protected against or immune to the disease for many years.

Against what diseases can we now immunize our children?

Children can now be immunized against the majority of childhood illnesses, including the following:
• Diphtheria
• Pertussis (whooping cough)
• Tetanus
• Polio
• Red measles (rubeola)
• German measles (rubella)
• Mumps
• *Hemophilus influenzae* meningitis

83

Due to advances in medical science, the 1st 7 of these diseases are not as deadly as they used to be, but it is still extremely important to continue to immunize children against them.

Why should we immunize our children against these diseases?

Until recently, many childhood diseases were on the way to becoming extinct, thanks largely to the availability of effective vaccines. Unfortunately, these optimistic statistics lured many people into a sense of false security. Since many adults remembered having these infections without complications (or not having them at all!), they felt that there was no urgency to getting their children immunized.

It is true that most of these diseases are less dangerous than they used to be, but severe cases may lead to serious or fatal complications. It is, therefore, extremely important for all parents to make sure that their children are adequately immunized. The greatest way that you can show your love for your child is to protect that child from preventable health problems. Immunizations are safe, effective, and relatively pain free, and they can go a long way in assuring your child a healthier adult life.

What are baby shots, and what do they do?

"Baby shots" are a series of immunizations given to an infant at 2, 4, and 6 months of age and again at 15 and 18 months of age. These series of injections are the 1st steps in providing lifelong immunity to specific illnesses.

The 1st baby shot is a combination shot called the DPT, which protects the child against diphtheria, pertussis (whooping cough), and tetanus. At the same time, the child is also given oral polio vaccine to begin the protection against polio. The DPT and polio vaccines are repeated at 4 and 6 months of age. The next immunization is given at approximately 15 months of age—another combination shot called the MMR. This shot protects the child against red measles, mumps, and rubella. At 18 months of age, the child receives a booster shot of DPT and oral polio vaccine.

It is critical that these shots are started at approximately 2 months of age and essential that the whole series of immunizations be given. Otherwise the child stands the risk of developing illness.

A new immunization is available and is recommended for children approximately 18 to 24 months of age. This shot, the *H. influenzae* vaccine, protects the child against contracting *Hemophilus influenzae* meningitis. (More about this particular illness in another section.)

84

Can't children have serious complications from the DPT shot?

There has been a great deal of discussion recently regarding the development of mental retardation and other complications in children who reacted adversely to the DPT shot, specifically the pertussis component. A study conducted in England did show that an extremely small number of children who had been immunized with the DPT vaccine did develop complications in later life.

This is a very critical point that must be explained to all parents. The risk of any serious consequences because you have had your child immunized is extremely small. In fact, your child stands a greater risk of developing complications from catching the disease than from the immunization itself.

Current medical procedure suggests that all physicians inform parents of the potential complications of the vaccinations themselves. He or she will also explain the child's risk of contracting these illnesses and developing complications such as deafness, mental retardation, or serious infections. Most parents will opt to take the relatively small risk of their child having a reaction to the vaccine rather than the larger risk of developing the disease.

Are there any side effects from these immunizations?

Probably 50% of children who receive the DPT shot will have some degree of side effects, most commonly localized swelling and tenderness at the site of the shot. This tenderness is caused not by the infection itself but by a reaction to the material in the immunization. The redness and swelling usually respond to applications of cold compresses to the area for about 15 minutes every couple of hours. The child will also feel more comfortable if given some acetaminophen drops at the same time.

About half the children also develop a slight fever (less than 102°) on the same day that they are vaccinated. This can be treated by giving acetaminophen drops. A better recommendation is to immediately give all children who receive the DPT shot a dose of acetaminophen drops and continue the drops every 4 hours for 24 to 48 hours.

A serious reaction to the DPT shots, such as a high fever, occurs in 1 out of 20 children. An even rarer occurrence is a child having a convulsion because of the high fever; this occurs in about 1 out of 1000 children. Since the pertussis vaccine is thought to be the major culprit in causing extremely high fever, I recommend that a child who has a history of developing fevers over 103° after 1 DPT shot, skip the pertussis vaccine and receive only the diphtheria and tetanus vaccines from that time on.

Does the MMR vaccine have any side effects?

The MMR vaccine is 1-shot protection against measles, mumps, and rubella. Some children develop a slight rash, fever, or swollen lymph nodes a week or so after receiving this shot. These reactions are mild and generally disappear within a few days. They are best treated by giving the child acetaminophen. A smaller number of children may have joint pain or stiffness anywhere from 1 to 10 weeks after receiving this vaccination. This side effect is also short-lived and generally goes away within a couple of days.

An extremely small number of children have developed an inflammation of the brain tissue called encephalitis after receiving the MMR vaccine. The chances of this happening are less than 1 in 1 million. Again, the risk of developing these side effects is small compared with the risk of more serious complications from measles or mumps.

MENINGITIS

I understand my child can be immunized against meningitis.

Hemophilus influenzae is a leading cause of serious bacterial meningitis in children under 5 years of age. Meningitis is an inflammation of the coating of the brain tissue and can lead to serious neurological problems. Approximately 12,000 cases are reported annually, and the mortality rate is about 5%; severe neurological problems can be observed in up to 25% of the survivors. Virtually all cases of *Hemophilus influenzae* meningitis among children are caused by strains of a germ called Type B. The Centers for Disease Control (CDC) has recommended a new immunization that protects your child against severe *Hemophilus influenzae* meningitis.

This vaccination has relatively few side effects and can potentially give long-lasting immunity to this particular disease. Because of its relatively low incidence of side effects, I recommend that children under 5 years of age, especially those between 18 and 24 months of age, receive this new vaccination. The side effects are similar to those of DPT and MMR. Slight fever and headache have been reported as well as local reactions of redness and tenderness around the injection site. The mild temperature elevation that frequently occurs will respond to acetaminophen. In over 60,000 doses given, only 1 serious side effect was reported: an acute allergic reaction that responded promptly to proper medication. Fevers higher than 101° have been reported in fewer than 1% of children receiving the vaccination.

DIPHTHERIA

What is diphtheria?

Diphtheria is caused by a bacteria that attacks the throat and causes a greyish membrane to form and grow. If this membrane gets too large, it can interfere with swallowing. In very severe cases, the membrane is so thick that air cannot get down the windpipe and suffocation results. This is why many children who developed diphtheria many years ago had to undergo a tracheostomy (the insertion of a breathing tube in the lower windpipe) to bypass the membrane until the infection cleared. Even though diphtheria can be cured, it may lead to serious (and sometimes fatal) complications.

A hundred years ago, diphtheria was a dreaded disease that claimed the lives of 15 out of every 100,000 Americans each year. As recently as the 1920s, diphtheria was a common affliction. The cases of diphtheria have dwindled because of the national immunization program supported by the American Medical Association, the American Academy of Family Physicians, and the American Academy of Pediatrics, but we continue to see occasional outbreaks in almost all parts of the country.

WHOOPING COUGH

What is whooping cough?

Whooping cough is an acute infectious disease caused by an organism known as *Hemophilus pertussis.* This germ attacks the breathing passages, causing a characteristic barking cough followed by whooping sounds at the end of the bouts of coughing. This whooping is the sound of the child gasping for air. Pertussis can produce serious complications including pneumonia and brain damage, especially in very young infants. Although whooping cough seldom occurs any more except in sporadic outbreaks, the dangerous nature of the disease reminds us that all children must continue to receive protection against it.

TETANUS

What is tetanus?

Tetanus is caused by the bacteria *Clostridium tetani,* commonly found in soil, dust, and the digestive tracts of humans and animals.

(This is why the manure of farm animals frequently contains the tetanus bacterium.)

The tetanus bacteria get into the body through a puncture wound, such as that caused by stepping on a rusty nail, or through a deep cut with a rusty knife or other object. Inside the body of an unimmunized person, the bacteria produce a strong poison called a toxin that causes painful swelling of the muscles, spasms, and stiffness. When the spasms and stiffness of the muscles affect the jaw, the infected person is unable to move the jaw—hence the common name of "lockjaw."

Even with advanced treatment available for tetanus, an unimmunized person who contracts the tetanus bacteria has about a 50-50 chance of dying from the infection. There is no lifetime vaccine against tetanus, so continued protection against it is mandatory for all children and adults. After the original series of 5 DPTs, a tetanus booster is recommended every 10 years.

POLIO

How common is polio today?

Polio epidemics may seem to be a thing of the past, but the disease is still a threat in many parts of the world. In fact in 1972, polio swept through a private boarding school in New England, striking 11 out of 129 students. Medical investigators found that only 1 who contracted polio had been vaccinated.

Polio is caused by a virus, and the disease has 2 stages. The 1st symptoms are a mild fever, headache, general weakness, and sometimes a sore throat—not unlike many of the viruses we contract today. About 3 to 5 days after this infection appears to be gone, the individual will come down with the symptoms again in a more serious form, and tremendous muscle weakness and/or paralysis will follow.

Most of us remember the iron lungs of the early 1900s when children had machines breathe for them because their breathing muscles had been totally paralyzed by the virus.

The chances of contracting polio from the oral vaccine are approximately 1 in 1 million: for every 1 million children vaccinated, only 1 stands a chance of developing the infection. An unimmunized child is much more likely to develop the infection if exposed to the virus.

MEASLES

Is there any difference between red measles and German measles?

Both measles infections are caused by viruses. In red measles (rubeola), a child will have a cough, a runny nose, conjunctivitis (red watery eyes), and a fever of 101° to 103°. This lasts about 3 days. When the fever starts to break, the child will develop a very red rash, starting on the face and spreading to the arms, legs, and torso. This rash tends to run together in huge patches and lasts around 7 to 10 days. Children who have the measles can spread the disease from the time they contract the fever until the rash is gone.

Rubella, or German measles, is usually a much milder infection. Children will not have any outstanding symptoms and may run only a low-grade fever. The 1st distinguishable sign of the disease is the formation of pinkish patches of rash on the body, not really as noticeable as the 3-day measle rash. Children with rubella or German measles often do not appear to be ill; the slight rash may be the only evidence that the child is sick. However, the child is infectious until the rash is gone. Rubella is often just a minor inconvenience for the child. The seriousness of this infection is if the child comes in contact with a woman in the early stages of pregnancy. A pregnant woman in her 1st trimester who is exposed to rubella has a significant chance of having a child with multiple abnormalities.

A frequent question concerns the incubation time for these diseases—the time between being exposed and actually coming down with the measles. In red measles, the child will start running a fever 1 to 2 weeks after coming in contact with an infected person. Rubella takes approximately 2 to 3 weeks to develop. If your child is *not* immunized and has come in contact with anyone with red or German measles, there is absolutely nothing you can do to prevent the child from coming down with the disease. At the 1st sign of a fever and rash, consult your physician to confirm the type of measles. Your physician will probably treat the child with acetaminophen (*not aspirin*) and will instruct you to keep the child indoors so as not to infect other children or pregnant women.

FIFTH DISEASE

What is fifth disease?

It is a viral infection that occurs in young children. The child will not appear to be ill but will, all of a sudden, develop a lacelike rash that looks as if the child has been slapped on each cheek. He or she will usually run a low-grade fever as the rash spreads to the arms and legs. The rash, usually apparent after the child has had a warm bath, lasts 7 to 10 days. There are few complications from this disease, and no treatment is necessary.

MUMPS

How serious is mumps?

Mumps is a childhood infection that occurs quite frequently in unimmunized children. It generally begins as a swelling of the parotid, or salivary, glands that sit under the angle of the jaw. The swelling begins 2 to 3 weeks after exposure and may affect 1 or both sides. Other symptoms of mumps are high fever, headache, and mild coughing or congestion.

If your child has a swelling in the neck and you want to decide if he or she has mumps, there is a test you can perform. If you can feel the angle of the jaw under the child's ear, the parotid gland is not swollen and your child does not have mumps. However, if the swelling obliterates the angle of the jawbone, the child most likely has the mumps.

Mumps generally runs its course in 5 to 7 days with few problems, but there can be some rare, serious side effects. We know that mumps in young men can involve the testicles. Young men who develop mumps that spreads to the testicles may become sterile. The virus that causes mumps may also cause a form of meningitis (an infection of the brain). If a child with mumps shows signs of a stiff neck in addition to the other symptoms, a physician should be contacted immediately.

Because mumps is caused by a virus, there is no specific treatment except to lower the fever, clear the congestion, and ease the pain of the swelling by applying warm compresses to either the swollen parotid glands or the testicles.

ASTHMA

What is asthma, and how is it treated in children?

Asthma occurs because the small air passages of the lung become tightened or constricted. This constriction can occur for several reasons:
- The muscles surrounding the bronchial tubes can tighten up, narrowing the tubes.
- The membrane that lines these bronchial tubes can swell, causing a narrowing of the opening.
- There can be an excessive amount of secretion or mucus that pours into the bronchial tubes, thus interfering with the flow of air.

Asthma occurs for many reasons, but probably in most children the asthmatic attack is triggered by an allergic reaction to something in the environment or substances such as house dust, pollens, mold spores, animal dander, or certain foods.

We also know that some children have asthmatic attacks for non-allergic reasons such as upper respiratory infections or bronchitis. In these cases, the asthma is cured once the original infection is treated.

The best way to avoid allergic attacks is to find out exactly what substances trigger them. In most children, an avoidance of these substances can significantly reduce the number of asthmatic attacks.

If your child has frequent asthmatic attacks that have to be treated by your physician, you may need to consult an allergy specialist who can do a series of tests, usually skin testing, to find out what substances or materials your child may be allergic to. Once identified, specific injections (hyposensitization shots) can be given that cause your child to build up a natural resistance to them.

The symptoms of asthma are different in every child but generally consist of difficulty in breathing, especially breathing out (a wheezing sound is created when the child breathes), and gasping for air. When any of these symptoms occur in your child, immediately consult your physician for treatment.

WHEN TO CALL THE DOCTOR

As a parent, how can I tell if my child is sick enough to call the doctor?

Even though I believe that parents' "sixth sense" is probably the best gauge, there are some guidelines you can use in determining whether or not you should call your physician. Among these are the following:
- If the child appears to be very weak, listless, and inactive
- If the child has labored breathing, even if you think it is just caused by a cold
- If the child cries and moans as if in pain for more than several hours
- If there are any complaints of ear pain
- If the child looks sick and is not eating or playing normally
- Any illness in a child under 2 months of age
- If a child's fever has continued for 3–4 days without any apparent cause
- If the child has any bleeding, such as through the rectum or mouth
- If the child has a convulsion

91

Although there may be other reasons to call your physician, you should certainly call him or her as soon as any of these appear. Use your own judgment. If you are not satisfied that your child is acting normally, then consult your physician.

5.

Common Problems of the Eyes

INTRODUCTION

Most of us tend to take our sense of sight for granted. Most people don't realize that the eyes are a special organ system of the body and need special attention and care. It is amazing that the same people who buckle their seat belts, eat properly, and get regular checkups neglect proper eye care. How many of you mow your grass and never consider wearing protective glasses? Do you get a yearly eye checkup whether you wear glasses or not? Most eye problems are subtle. They tend to come on slowly and give very few symptoms. But if left unnoticed and untreated, many of these subtle symptoms can lead to permanent blindness. That is why it is strongly recommended that we have yearly eye examinations to detect any potential problem within the eye early enough so that it can be corrected.

CHILDREN'S EYESIGHT

Are there any special problems dealing with children's eyesight?

The most difficult problem with children's eyesight is that very few of them will complain when things are not right. We adults have certain standards by which to gauge our eyesight. We can tell from day to day if our sight is changing because we know from experience over the years what our sight ought to be. Children lack this experience and, therefore, believe that what they are seeing is what everyone else is seeing.

Parents will ask their children if they are having any problems with their eyes, but the children will answer no because they feel that the images they see are normal, even if that is not the case. This becomes a critical problem when we consider that a majority of children's learning problems in school stem from problems with vision.

Never rely on your child's telling you that his or her vision is okay. Children's eyes should be checked after they reach the age of 3 and again before they enter school. After that, their eyes should be checked at least every few years to make sure that normal vision is maintained.

What are some of the more common problems that children have with their eyes?

The most common vision problems of children affect their ability to see clearly and sharply. If a child has myopia (nearsightedness), he or she will see close objects much clearer than objects at a distance. If a child has hyperopia (farsightedness), objects will be clear at a distance but will become more blurred and unfocused at close range. Some children will have an astigmatism: objects are distorted and look as if they are superimposed on each other.

Fortunately, all of these conditions can be helped through corrective lenses. But if the problems go undetected, a child may have difficulty in reading, writing, and communicating properly.

I have been told that my child has a lazy eye.

Each eye has the ability to look in all directions—up, down, and sideways—because of special muscles attached to the eye. When these muscles contract or relax, the eye is turned 1 way or the other. Through an amazing system of coordinating the muscles of both eyes, the eyes generally move in unison.

In children, 1 or more of these muscles can be underdeveloped or weak, causing 1 eye to lag behind and appear not to move and focus with the other. Almost all children are born with eye muscles that are not as strong as they eventually will be, and over the first 6 to 9 months of life, the eye muscles should develop enough strength so that the child moves the eyes in unison. If 1 eye continually turns inward or outward or lags behind the other, a proper ophthalmic evaluation should be given before the child's 1st birthday. Many weak eye muscle problems can be corrected through the use of eye-strengthening exercises. However, when they become so severe as to potentially affect the proper development of the good eye, corrective surgery may be necessary.

Although operating on the eye seems frightening or even dangerous, it is a safe procedure when performed by a well-trained surgeon. And performing this type of surgery can save your child a multitude of vision problems in the future.

If my child took the eye chart test and had 20/20 vision, does that mean that his or her eyesight is normal?

Not necessarily. The screening eye chart test is a good way to tell whether or not vision is within normal ranges, but you must understand that this test misses many of the potential problems that both children and adults can have. Problems with near vision such as reading, eye coordination, and the ability to focus at short distances are among the many problems that cannot be identified through a routine eye chart test.

Using the screening test is perfectly acceptable in evaluating a child's sight prior to entering school, but it is recommended that a more thorough medical examination of the eyes be undertaken to rule out any other problems.

Should children have 20/20 vision?

As you know, the numbers 20 over 20 are used to describe "normal" vision. The figure 20/20 means that at a distance of 20' the individual can read the line on the chart marked 20. If at 20' the numbers at the line 20 cannot be read and only the larger numbers can be read, the vision would change to 20 over 30 or 20 over 40. The higher the lower numbers gets, the more indication there is that sight is not normal.

Remember that very young children do not have 20/20 vision because the eye mechanism has not developed to the point of having "normal" adult sight. However, some time between the ages of 5 and 7, all children should begin to develop 20/20 vision. If your child has taken the screening eye chart test and has been found to have something other than 20/20 vision, he or she should have a thorough evaluation by an eye specialist. This does not mean that the child's sight is poor and that glasses need to be prescribed; it does mean that an ocular problem *may* be present. Many times a more thorough evaluation will show normal eyes, and the eye specialist will simply wait until the child's eyes mature before evaluating the need for glasses.

AGING AND EYESIGHT

Does sight change as you get older?

It's not always the case, but most people will find some change in their eyesight as they get older. This is because of the changes that take place in the structure of the eye. As we get older, the water content in the lens of the eye tends to decrease and alters the configuration of the lens. The most common change with the lens is referred to as pres-

95

byopia, which means a decrease in the eye's ability to focus at close range. This normal process of aging is the reason why most adults need corrective lenses at some time.

There are also times when vision will actually improve with age: it is not uncommon for some nearsighted adults to find that as they get older they can actually read better if they take their glasses off. Other people will find that their ability to see at a distance will actually improve with age. Any change, however, that takes place in your vision should be reported to your eye specialist and thoroughly evaluated.

SERIOUS SYMPTOMS

If I am having a problem with my eyes, how can I tell if it's serious enough to see a physician?

We all have occasional episodes of irritation when the eyes sting or burn or are a little red for a short period of time. But if these symptoms persist longer than 24 hours, contact your physician.

Without question, any unusual pain in the eye should be reported immediately. Pain, especially when associated with redness, is a warning sign that something significant has occurred within the eye. Any sudden change in vision, such as blurry vision or seeing double, should be reported immediately to your physician.

INFECTIONS OF THE EYELID

What causes irritation of the eyelids?

Your eyelids contain hair follicles located at the margins or borders. These hair follicles lie deep in your eyelids, and the hair or eyelash grows outward. The small glands at the base of the eyelash are very common sites of potential infection.

A person with an eyelash infection (called blepharitis) usually has some local irritation and burning around the lid. Lid margins can become red and form some crusty material, which may cause the lids to stick together, especially in the mornings. If the infection continues without treatment, loss of eyelashes may result, and the lid margins may swell. People with blepharitis should report the condition to their physician as soon as possible. Treatment consists of a combination of cleaning and antibiotics. Each morning, the lid margins should be carefully cleaned with either a cotton applicator or a cotton swab soaked in warm water. Once the crust has been removed, a cotton swab can be used to apply a special antibiotic ointment. Because the infection is generally caused by the staphylococcus bacteria, the combination of a thorough cleaning and antibiotic ointment usually suffices to cure the condition. The individual should be advised that when the treatment is started, the ointment should be applied 4 times a day and response is usually not evident for 1 to 2 weeks.

What causes a sty?

A single sty, or hordeolum, is generally caused by a bacterial infection of a gland in the upper or lower eyelid. The infection gets in the base of the gland and causes the typical signs of infection: pain, swelling, redness, and a feeling of warmth. Along with these symptoms comes the formation of a very tender infected nodule or lump. The sty may point externally (directly through the skin), internally (to the inner portion of the eye), or to the base of the eyelash.

The treatment of sties consists of time and the application of hot compresses. Washcloths placed in hot water and then applied to the sty for 15 minutes, 4 times a day, will usually bring it to a head. When the sty is pointing in toward the eye, antibiotic drops to the eye help protect the eye when the infection ruptures.

Occasionally a sty becomes so severe that improvement is hastened by nicking it with a sterile needle when it comes to a head. *Warning: This should never be done by you. It should be done only by your physician.*

What causes a hard knot to form in the eyelid?

When a bacterial infection gets into the deep gland of the eyelid (the meibomian gland), a chalazion may be formed. In the very early stages, a chalazion is difficult to distinguish from a sty since it can have the same symptoms of redness, tenderness, and swelling. However, a chalazion does not drain spontaneously, and the infection generally goes away on its own, leaving a hard nodule.

Approximately 50% of these chalazions will spontaneously disappear within a month or so. If it does not go away on its own, or if it becomes cosmetically unacceptable, you should see an ophthalmologist (a trained eye specialist) to discuss removing it.

RED EYE AND PINKEYE

What causes a red eye?

The causes of a red eye range from very mild infections to very serious sight-threatening conditions such as acute angle-closure glaucoma. The cause of your red eye should be determined by a physician.

As I said before, if you suddenly develop a red eye that is accompanied by pain, contact your physician. He or she will want to examine you fairly soon to determine if this is a minor problem that can be treated very simply or an indication of a more serious underlying problem.

What is pinkeye?

The conjunctiva is the membrane that covers the white portion of the eyeball and the inner part of the eyelids. Pinkeye, also called conjunctivitis, occurs when the conjunctiva becomes infected with a virus or bacteria. The infection makes the eye look red or pink, and can also produce the sensation of grittiness—as if you had sand in your eye. Most people with conjunctivitis will also experience a discharge of fluid or pus, which will make the eye stick and mat together.

Pinkeye is generally a very harmless but highly contagious condition. Pinkeye can cause a great deal of discomfort and is often treated with antibiotic eyedrops. In many cases, however, it will clear up by itself in 7 to 10 days.

How can I keep from spreading pinkeye?

Pinkeye is so contagious that the chances of its spreading from 1 eye to the other are greater than 75%. Pinkeye can also spread rapidly through a family or through a classroom within just a few days.

To help keep this infection from spreading, you should observe the following precautions:
• Avoid touching or rubbing the infected eye; don't touch the uninfected eye after you have touched the infected eye. If your child has pinkeye, make sure you wash your hands thoroughly with soap and water after applying medication or touching your child around the eye for any reason.
• Wash your hands thoroughly with soap and water throughout the day, and keep from touching your eyes or your face.
• Wash any discharge from your eye twice a day using disposable paper towels, facial tissues, or towels that are immediately placed in a basin soaked with antiseptic.
• Wash any cloth towels, washclothes, or linens you may have used separate from the rest of your family's laundry. Hot water and detergent are the best for washing.
• If you have pinkeye, don't use your contact lenses or eye makeup until the eye is totally healed.

SUBCONJUNCTIVAL HEMORRHAGE

What causes the sudden appearance of a red spot in the eye?

The sudden appearance of a red spot or red blotch in the eye may be due to a subconjunctival hemorrhage—ruptured blood vessels in the white portion of your eye. Often these blood vessels rupture because of trauma—rubbing the eye, a scratch on the eyeball, a blow by a rock or baseball. Subconjunctival hemorrhages can occur spontaneously in people with hypertension and arteriosclerosis and can also be caused by straining that occurs during vomiting, coughing, sneezing, or having a difficult bowel movement. Or they may happen for no apparent reason.

The immediate treatment for these hemorrhages consists of ice cold compresses applied to the closed eye for 10 minutes, 4 times a day. These compresses should be continued for approximately 2 to 3 days; after the 3rd day, alternate cold compresses with warm ones.

Although they look terrible, the vast majority of these hemorrhages will spontaneously resolve. (You'll find that the beefy red hemorrhages will begin to turn yellow and greenish colors before they totally disappear.)

Subconjunctival hemorrhages generally do not interfere at all with eyesight because they appear on the white portion of the eye, the conjunctiva, and have nothing to do with the pupil.

FOREIGN SUBSTANCES

What should I do if I think I may have a foreign substance in my eye?

Almost anything can get in the eyes. Some of the most common foreign bodies that end up in the eye are sand, pieces of metal flying off machinery, small pieces of wood, eyelashes, particles of eyeliner or mascara, and different chemicals.

If you suspect something has gotten into your eye, immediately flush it out thoroughly with cold water. Often the foreign body has not embedded itself in the eye, and this procedure will wash the foreign body away. The eye may be irritated for 24 hours after this, but it generally will require no specific treatment by your physician. If, however, you experience persistent pain in the eye even after flushing, you should consult your physician immediately.

Remember that the best way to avoid getting foreign materials in your eye is to *always* wear protective glasses especially when working around machinery, or mowing the grass.

How will my physician get a foreign body out of my eye?

When you go to your physician because you feel that something is in your eye, a thorough examination will be performed. Your vision will be tested to see if there is any change because of a possible foreign body. Then your physician will thoroughly examine your eye with the help of a penlight and ophthalmoscope. Many times the foreign body can be detected through these simple measures. If your physician cannot see the foreign body, he or she will place a special staining material in the eye. This fluorescent stain is placed in the eye, which is then observed with a cobalt penlight. Normally the eye lining will not pick up this fluorescent stain, but if a foreign body is in the eye and has scratched or embedded itself in the eye surface, that will be marked by the fluorescent stain.

The physician will then remove the foreign body after placing a drop of anesthetizing fluid on your eyeball. Then the eye will be examined again to see if there is a scratch or abrasion. If the foreign body left a scratch, the eye must be allowed to heal.

The optimum way to do this is to put a special antibiotic cream in the eye and then patch the eye for 1 or 2 days. Most patients will be asked to return to the physician's office after that period of time for reexamination and restain of the eye.

The eye has a tremendous ability to heal itself. If the foreign body is removed soon, the eye should sustain no permanent damage.

I got a piece of metal in my eye, and my physician told me I also had a rust ring.

If you have ever left a piece of metal on a wet counter top and come back 2 or 3 days later, you found that the counter top had a ring of rust left on it. That was because the moisture of the counter top interacted with the metal, leaving the rust. The same process takes place if a piece of metal (no matter how small) is left in the eye for any length of time. Even if the foreign body is removed, a rust stain will remain on the cornea. This rust stain must be removed, or it will become a permanent part of the cornea. Fortunately, this can be done simply and painlessly by an eye specialist, and the portion of the eye lining that has been involved is treated with antibiotic ointment and patching as described before.

What is a corneal abrasion?

The lining of the eyeball and especially the cornea are tremendously sensitive. Corneal abrasions, or scratches, are some of the most painful conditions that people experience. These abrasions can vary from small hairline scratches to massive scratches extending across the whole eye.

Whether the abrasion on your eye is large or small, it needs to be seen by a physician and adequately treated.

The 1st thing your physician will do is to evaluate your eye and the extent of the damage and then place some drops in the eye that will deaden the pain. Then antibiotic ointment and a patch will be applied. Depending upon the extent of the scratch, the eye will generally heal itself within 1 to 3 days. These types of scratches must be followed closely by your physician to make sure that they heal properly without scarring. Any scarring that occurs on the eyeball, especially the pupil, could significantly reduce your vision in the future.

SPECIAL VISION PROBLEMS

What causes spots before the eyes?

A common eye complaint is "spots before the eyes." To understand what causes this, we have to look at the basic anatomy of the eye itself. Behind the lens of the eye is an inner chamber filled with a jellylike fluid; this vitreous fluid is extremely important in the proper transmission of light and images to the back part of the eye or retina.

Sometimes (especially as people get older) this jellylike fluid can clump together, forming an opacity—usually seen as a floating spot. If these spots move as you turn your eye (as is usually the case), they are not serious and do not mean that you are going to lose your eyesight. With time, these opacities tend to fall through the vitreous to the lower portion of the inner chamber and out of your line of sight.

If, however, these spots before your eyes become lightning flashes or a feeling as if the "curtain is coming down in front of your eyes," you should consult your physician immediately. This sensation could indicate that the back portion of the eye or the retina is beginning to tear away, forming a retinal detachment.

What is a retinal detachment?

The back portion of the inner chamber of the eye is lined with a specialized material called the retina. Through the functioning of the retina, light is transferred into electrical impulses and sight is achieved. A retinal detachment occurs when a portion of this retina separates from the back part of the eye. Retinal detachments generally begin with a small opening that allows the vitreous fluid to flow in and push the retina from the back portion of the eye.

People who experience a retinal detachment often notice a sudden shower of the vitreous "floaters" I have described. This is caused by

101

blood cells from the torn retina bleeding into the vitreous fluid. Over the next few hours, the individual generally complains of flashes of light, until finally there is a feeling as if a curtain has fallen over the eyes.

Retinal detachments are medical emergencies. Anyone who experiences these symptoms should see a physician immediately; if a detachment has occurred, the person will probably be hospitalized without delay. Retinal detachments can easily be treated with modern advances in laser surgery where the laser beam is pinpointed to the tear and causes a scarring of the retina, which reattaches it to the posterior portion of the eye.

Why does my eye physician check the pressure in my eyes?

In each eye a certain pressure is maintained within the inner structures. The measurement of this intraocular pressure is important because if the pressure becomes too great, the individual could develop a condition known as glaucoma. Tonometry is the determination of the intraocular pressure by means of an instrument called a Schiötz tonometer. Tonometry begins by placing a mild anesthetic on the eyeball. Then, with the person's eye open, the tonometer is gently placed on the outer surface of the cornea, and through a series of weights and measurements, a correct measurement of the pressure within the eye is made.

Ophthalmologists (eye specialists) have a more sophisticated instrument that can measure the pressure within your eye with a machine that blows a puff of air against the eyeball; the amount of pressure is measured by calculating the resistance to the puff of air. Normal pressure within an eyeball is generally between 12 and 25 mm of mercury pressure. When the pressure rises above 25 mm in either eye, your physician will become concerned that you could be suffering from glaucoma.

What is glaucoma?

Glaucoma is a condition in which the pressure in the eyes builds up to such an extent that normal functioning and sight become impossible. The National Society to Prevent Blindness reports hundreds of thousands of Americans have glaucoma, which is the 3rd major cause of blindness in the United States.

Within the eye is a mechanism for a continuous production of fluid in the anterior portion of the eye, in other words, the portion of the eye in front of the lens. There is also a mechanism called Schlemm's canal for continuous drainage of the fluid.

Whenever there is some resistance to the outward flow through this canal, a pressure is built up in the anterior portion of the eye. The greater the resistance to flow, the higher the pressure in the eye. And the higher the pressure, the greater the chance of loss of normal vision.

The important fact regarding the diagnosis of glaucoma is that it can be medically controlled *if* it is detected early. The problem with glaucoma is that it is an insidious disease; the symptoms and impairment in vision occur gradually. Some people, as they get older, feel that their sight is getting bad just because of age when in fact they have developed glaucoma. When your physician checks the pressure in your eyes and finds it to be abnormally high, the diagnosis of glaucoma may be made. Your physician will then place you on medication to put into your eyes every day to lower the pressure in the eyes by increasing the drainage of fluids from the eye chambers. As the pressure is lowered, the chance of permanent eye damage is reduced.

Why do some people with glaucoma suffer a sudden onset?

There is another type of glaucoma, acute angle-closure glaucoma, which is much less common. In this particular form, the canal is abruptly closed, causing a rapid rise in the internal eye pressure. This causes symptoms that are not found in the slower onset glaucoma: feeling sudden pain, becoming nauseous, or seeing halos around lights. When the eye is examined during an acute attack of glaucoma, it is generally red and teary with a hazy cornea. The eye is extremely firm to pressure.

In acute angle-closure glaucoma, physicians must institute treatment immediately or the rapid buildup in pressure can cause permanent damage to the optic nerve and endanger sight.

What causes cataracts?

The eye acts on the same principle as a camera. There is an opening (the pupil), a lens, and a developing film called the retina. The lens of the eye performs the same function as the lens of the camera—focusing the light images on the back portion of the eye. The lens is a colorless structure made up of specialized tissue, and its function is to focus light rays on the retina. To focus these rays properly, the lens will actually become fatter or thinner, depending upon the intensity of the light.

The lens consists of about 60% water. As people get older, the water content of the lens can change dramatically, causing the lens to become cloudy or opaque; this clouding of the lens is known as cataract formation. Occurring most commonly in older people, it is present in some degree in almost everyone over 60. Most cataracts occur in both eyes, although the rate of development can differ.

The chief complaint caused by cataracts is a decrease in visual acuity. Cataracts in the early stages can be seen only by special light instruments of the physician, but as the cataracts become more opaque, or cloudy, they can be seen by the naked eye.

The speed at which the vision deteriorates because of cataracts is difficult to determine. In some people, the cataracts will form rather quickly, and vision will deteriorate accordingly. However, many people can have cataracts for years and years without a significant change in their ability to see.

Cataracts should be closely followed by your physician. Most physicians believe that cataracts should not be operated on until vision is significantly impaired. At that point, the opaque lens can be removed through cataract surgery and replaced with either a contact lens or a specialized artificial lens. Cataract surgery is perhaps the most common surgery performed on the eye today. In the skilled hands of an eye surgeon, it is a safe, successful procedure. Many people whose sight had been significantly impaired by cataracts have recovered a great portion of sight through surgery.

6.

Health Problems of the Ears and Nose

HEARING

How does the ear work?

One of the most remarkable organs in the body is the ear. It is amazing to think that a noise up to several miles away can be instantaneously transmitted into the brain and distinguished as to its cause and location.

The earlobe or outer ear functions as a funnel where sound is reflected into the canal leading to the eardrum. As the sound hits the thin, flexible tissue of the eardrum, it creates a vibration at approximately the same frequency the sound makes. Behind the eardrum is the small chamber called the middle ear. Here, a combination of 3 tiny bones called the ossicles act as a unit and conduct vibrations from the eardrum to the inner ear.

These delicate bones vibrating freely in the middle ear not only transmit the vibrations but actually increase the power of the sound waves. The vibrations from the bones are transmitted to the plate at the opening of the inner ear, which in turn vibrates, causing a liquid substance in the inner ear to vibrate. This liquid substance is carried through a series of circular canals—the cochlea—which is actually shaped like a snail. Each fluid-filled canal is lined by a fine membrane. The small hairs of the membrane protrude into the liquid medium, and as the vibrations are carried through the liquid, they stimulate tiny hairs. The hairs are, in turn, attached to nerve tissue, which creates an electrical impulse when stimulated. Each smaller nerve then grows to form a larger and larger nerve until eventually the major hearing, or auditory, nerve is formed. The electrical impulse is carried through the auditory nerve into the brain tissue where it is translated into the perception and identification of the sound.

So, a bell ringing around the corner sets the air in motion that vibrates against the eardrum, that in turn vibrates the small bones of the middle ear, and that vibrates the liquid medium of the inner ear and stimulates the small hearing nerves, which carry the electrical impulses to the brain. Therefore, hearing is the changing of sound waves to electrical impulses in the brain.

HEARING PROBLEMS

What is a hearing impairment?

Simply stated, a hearing impairment is an inability to hear speech and other sounds clearly. The inability to hear speech and other sounds loudly enough is considered a loss of hearing sensitivity, or a hearing loss.

For some people, it may be an inability to hear speech and music clearly, even if the sound is sufficiently loud. What is heard may be similar to garbled speech from a radio with a broken speaker. This is known as an impairment in speech discrimination.

For still others, hearing impairment is an inability to understand or use speech in communication, even though speech is sufficiently loud and can be heard clearly. This is called an impairment in language reception.

How common are hearing impairments?

Hearing impairments are probably the most frequently reported disorders in the numerous surveys conducted by the United States Public Health Service; 6 out of every 100 people reported some kind of hearing problem, but only 5 out of 100 people reported a visual problem. Statistics show that approximately 16 million Americans have trouble hearing in 1 or both ears; 3 out of every 100 school children suffer from some degree of hearing problem; and 30 out of every 100 people 65 years of age or older have trouble hearing.

What are some types of hearing problems?

We have already discussed the different varieties of hearing impairment, such as hearing loss, difficulty hearing spoken words, and difficulty understanding and using the spoken word. There are also classifications of hearing impairment based on the location of the problem within the hearing mechanism.

106

A conductive hearing loss occurs when the sound is not conducted sufficiently through the ear canal, the eardrum, or the small bones in the middle ear. This can be caused by blockage, damage to the outer or middle structures, or excessive fluid behind the eardrum.

A sensorineural type of hearing loss occurs when there is damage to or malformation of the structures of the inner ear, specifically the auditory nerve that transmits impulses from the ear to the brain.

Many people have signs or symptoms of both conductive and sensorineural type losses and are categorized as having "mixed" hearing impairment.

The final type of hearing impairment occurs when there is damage or destruction to the tissues in the brain that translate the sense of hearing. This is known as a central hearing loss.

What causes some people to have problems with their hearing?

Hearing impairments can stem from a variety of causes. Some people will have permanent hearing damage from exposure to loud noises. This is common in those who for years have worked around loud machinery, have listened to too-loud music, or have suddenly been exposed to an extremely loud noise, such as a shotgun blast or an explosion. Some people inherit permanent hearing loss.

Aging creates changes in the middle ear and the inner ear and in the auditory nerve. So aging, too, becomes a possible cause of hearing impairment. Women tend to lose lower frequency hearing while men tend to lose higher frequency hearing.

Certain medications, such as strong antibiotics, taken for too long a period of time can damage the auditory nerve and result in a loss of hearing.

Some people develop tumors in the ear that can either block or destroy the ear's normal functioning.

Others can have a loss of hearing because of infections they have contracted. A common example of this is the deafness in children caused by measles infections. Many children also develop difficulty with hearing because of repeated infections in the middle ear itself. As noted earlier, the 3 small bones of the middle ear must function in unison, and this can only be accomplished when there is no fluid surrounding them.

A common cause of nonpermanent hearing loss is a blockage of the outer canal. Large wax buildups can create a barrier to the normal transmission of sound waves to the eardrum. This is one of the only types of hearing loss that can be permanently corrected.

Should certain people have their hearing checked frequently?

It is very important to screen and evaluate the hearing in newborn infants. If we rely on the normal ways to detect decreased hearing—inability to hear or respond to the spoken voice—we will be unable to detect hearing difficulties in many infants. This is particularly true for infants born with a high risk of developing hearing impairment: a history of other children in the family with hearing impairments; rubella or other fetal infections during pregnancy; obvious birth defects involving the ear, nose, or throat; and children born prematurely.

It is also important to screen and evaluate the hearing of children as they enter school. The inability to hear properly contributes to learning difficulties and failure to adjust to the school environment. Early identification of hearing problems *before* a child gets into the school years creates a better educational environment and reduces the chances of a child's being mistakenly diagnosed as having a learning disorder.

I also recommend that any adults who notice a change in their hearing should see a physician and have their hearing evaluated. Too many adults lose out on a great portion of their later years because they do not take the time to have their hearing checked or they are too embarrassed to admit that they could have a problem.

Why can't I hear well when I have a bad cold?

Remember that it is very important for the small bones in the middle ear to vibrate freely. When people develop severe colds, they also develop a great deal of congestion that blocks the eustachian tube, the normal passageway between the middle ear and the outside environment. When the eustachian tube is congested, pressure builds up in the middle ear and causes increased fluid formation behind the eardrum. So, fluid surrounds the 3 small bones and prevents their vibrating freely. This obviously cuts down on the transmission of sound from the middle ear to the inner ear, which results in a decrease in hearing. Once the fluid leaves the middle ear, the bones will resume their normal functioning, and your hearing should return to normal.

EAR INFECTIONS

How common is ear infection in adults?

The most common cause of adult ear pain is external otitis, an infection of the outer ear canal.

The occurrence of external otitis, or swimmer's ear, peaks during the summer months and is generally caused by infection from the *Pseudomonas* organisms found in swimming pools and lakes.

An adult with swimmer's ear has pain in the ear that gets particularly acute when the outer ear is either touched or tugged. People with outer ear infections will generally complain of itching along with pain, but there is usually no fever associated with it.

The treatment of an outer ear infection depends upon a correct diagnosis and the application of antibiotic ear drops that control the pain and itching within 2 or 3 days.

What causes middle ear infections?

Middle ear infections are referred to as otitis media. *Otitis* refers to the inflammation of the ear and *media* refers to the middle section of the ear behind the eardrum. Middle ear infections generally start by blockage of the eustachian tube, which connects the middle ear to the back of the throat. When the eustachian tube becomes blocked, fluids will accumulate behind the eardrum. We can tell when the eustachian tube is blocked by the sensation of popping and clicking in the ear and a full feeling, which may be associated with a decreased ability to hear. If this fluid stays in the ear too long, it can become infected, causing a pressure buildup and pain.

Middle ear infections are exceptionally common in children but also occur in adults. They must be treated with antibiotics. The most common bacteria creating the infection are pneumococcus, streptococcus, and staphylococcus. Depending upon your age and the seriousness of the infection, different types of antibiotics may be prescribed. The antibiotics will cause a decrease in the infection and a decrease in the swelling around the eustachian tube which will help the middle ear to drain.

My child had a severe earache, and all of a sudden the ear began to drain. What can cause this?

Middle ear infections, otitis media, can create a tremendous amount of pressure behind the eardrum. Occasionally this pressure tries to relieve itself, and because it cannot get through the eustachian tube, it will create its own opening through the eardrum. These are generally small openings and allow the pressure to be reduced, causing the sudden drainage. This is referred to as chronic otitis media.

Don't panic if this happens to your child. This does not mean that the child's hearing will be permanently lost nor that severe hearing problems will occur in the future. It does mean, however, that the infection needs to be treated right away. Never put drops in a child's ear that has begun to drain because of the possibility that the drainage is caused by a ruptured eardrum. Drops placed in the ear of a ruptured eardrum can seep through the rupture into the middle ear and cause problems.

Once the infection has cleared, the small opening will heal itself fairly quickly. There are, however, some ruptures of the eardrum that do not heal and a special graft will have to be placed over the opening.

TINNITUS (RINGING IN EARS)

What causes ringing in my ears?

A persistent ringing in 1 or both ears is referred to as tinnitus. According to the American Council of Otolaryngology, nearly 36 million Americans suffer from this condition, which ranges from periodic, annoying ringing to a persistent ringing that is not only annoying but can interfere with a normal lifestyle. More than 7 million Americans are affected so severely that they cannot lead normal lives.

There are many possible causes for subjective tinnitus, a noise that only the patient can hear. Tinnitus may result from something as simple as a plug of wax in the ear, but it can also be a symptom of more serious middle ear problems—infection, a hole in the eardrum, or an accumulation of fluid. Many of these problems are also associated with a decrease or loss of hearing.

Ringing in the ears can also be caused by allergies, high or low blood pressure, tumors affecting the nerve leading to the ear, or diabetes or thyroid problems.

What is the most common cause of tinnitus?

Probably the most common cause of ringing in the ears involves the auditory nerve. The health of this nerve is important for normal hearing, and any damage to it usually brings about a hearing loss and constant vibration sound. Damage to the auditory nerve generally accompanies the natural aging process.

Another, although less frequent, cause of damage to the nerve is constant bombardment by loud noises, such as industrial noise or loud music. Even though the normal aging process is the most common reason for ringing in the ears, this condition can and does occur in young people. If you need a good excuse to convince your teenagers to turn down the music, make sure you tell them that it can, and often does, cause permanent damage.

Is there any cure for tinnitus?

The most important thing to remember about tinnitus is that a thorough evaluation is necessary before determining the specific treatment. When your physician undertakes a thorough evaluation, he or she will be looking for specific causes that are correctable. If a plug of wax is present, it will be removed; if the ear is infected or fluid has accumulated, that problem will be appropriately treated.

However, since the most common cause of tinnitus is damage to the middle ear or the auditory nerve, there will be no cure for most people who suffer from this (especially the elderly).

Although there is no cure, can anything be done to lessen the annoying ringing?

There are many do's and don'ts that can lessen its severity. The auditory (hearing) system is a delicate, sensitive mechanism of the human body. The auditory nerve, especially, is extremely sensitive to any stimulation of the nervous system. Therefore, it is desirable to make every effort to:

- Reduce any underlying anxiety, especially the anxiety that is associated with the ringing itself. Although the noise is sometimes maddening, it is not life-threatening; your ability to control the nervousness it creates will help reduce the severity of the ringing.
- Get adequate rest, avoid overfatigue, and take frequent naps, if appropriate. Fatigue is a stress that seems to increase the intensity and the frequency of the ringing.
- Avoid anything that will increase the stimulation of the nerve, such as caffeine and nicotine. People with ringing in the ears should avoid colas, coffee, and chocolates.
- Stop worrying about the noise. Tinnitus will not cause you to go deaf or make you "lose your mind" as long as you are able to control your response to it. Getting your attention off the noises and onto other things will help reduce the noise and lessen your anxiety.

HEARING AIDS AND THE AGED

Why do older people require hearing aids?

A common cause of hearing loss in people over 65 is a condition called presbycusis. This hearing loss occurs during the natural aging of the middle ear and the auditory nerve. The degree to which the hearing loss affects the individual is related to any preexisting hearing deficit that the individual may have had. For instance, people who have had a lot of ear infections or chronic exposure to noise will probably experience a greater hearing loss during the normal aging process.

A common misconception is that individuals who are 65 and suffer from presbycusis cannot benefit from amplification through the use of hearing aids. Even though this is a sensorineural hearing loss, hearing aids have been found to have a significant impact on the ability of these people to understand normal communication.

Of the estimated 1 million hearing aids sold in the United States each year, over 50% were sold to people over 65 years of age. Anyone over 65 who experiences some degree of hearing loss should have a proper evaluation, including an audiological test. With this test, your doctor or hearing specialist can better assess the benefits you might achieve from a hearing aid. Never assume that your hearing loss is not correctable, no matter what your age.

RUPTURE OF THE EARDRUM

Is it possible for me to rupture my own eardrum?

Yes. A common mistake people make is to try to clean out their ears by placing a cotton swab or other object deep into the ear canal. This should *never* be done. The distance between your outer ear and the eardrum is short, and in some people, even inserting cotton swabs can potentially rupture the eardrum. Also, the ear canal itself is extremely sensitive to this type of trauma and will bleed easily.

Never place anything into your ear. If you do, you will not only experience pain, but you could rupture your tympanic membrane causing potential hearing problems.

NOSEBLEED

What is the best way to treat a nosebleed?

Nosebleeds can be divided into different categories depending upon where the bleeding begins. About 90% of all nosebleeds are caused by rupture of the small blood vessels toward the inside tip of the nose. These nosebleeds are generally controllable by immediately pinching the tip of the nose and holding the pressure for 15 to 30 minutes. Ice packs can also be placed over the tip of the nose.

If you develop a nosebleed, perform these simple techniques immediately. Lie down, remain calm, pinch the nose, and use the ice packs. Generally after 30 minutes, the nosebleed will subside. If you have no further bleeding, try a nasal spray such as Neo-Synephrine (1%), but only apply it 2 to 3 times a day and only for 2 to 3 days. If the nosebleed continues, repeat the above procedures. If it still has not stopped, consult your physician.

ALLERGY OR COLD?

My nose constantly runs. Does that mean that I could have an allergy?

Rhinitis, a runny nose, is a frequent complaint. Rhinitis may be caused by allergies if it seems to occur only during certain seasons of the year. For instance, if you have a lot of drippage and drainage during the spring and fall, it's a good possibility that you are allergic to something in the environment during those times of the year. If you have constant rhinitis throughout the year, you could be allergic to something in your everyday environment such as mold and mildew.

Rhinitis is a problem that, if it is not severe, can be treated with any number of over-the-counter decongestant/antihistamines, which can decrease the runny nose and control the symptoms without much difficulty. A word of caution: Many people will turn to nasal sprays to stop the drippage and drainage and forget that too-frequent usage of them can cause harm.

NASAL SPRAY

Can you become addicted to nasal spray?

A nasal spray stops the drainage by shrinking the mucous membranes of the lining of the nasal cavity. That's all well and good if it is only used for 2 to 3 days. Any further use of the spray can cause a chemical irritation in the lining and actually increase the amount of drainage. Remember, this new drainage is not caused by the allergy or cold but by the irritation of the chemicals. Some people, however, feel that their colds or allergies have gotten worse and, therefore, use more and more nasal spray. The more they use, the more the nose drips, and these people can actually become addicted to nasal sprays.

Addiction to nasal sprays is typified by people who say that they have to use the sprays almost every hour to clear nasal congestion. It is difficult to get these people off nasal sprays once they have become addicted. They are not easily convinced that the nasal spray, not an underlying cold or infection, is causing the difficulty in breathing.

7.

Health Problems of the Lungs

THE LUNGS

How do the lungs work?

The body's ability to take in oxygen from the air and to expel potentially dangerous gases is a fascinating process. The breathing mechanism can be compared to a tree. There is a large trunk, called the trachea, leading down into the lung tissue. The trachea then branches off into 2 rather large branches, 1 going into each lung. These branches, or bronchi, then further divide, like the limbs of a tree, until they finally reach the outside of the lung tissue, the alveoli.

Air travels down through the trachea, through the bronchial tree, and into the lung tissue where the exchange of oxygen for carbon dioxide takes place. When the air that you breathe in travels all the way to the alveoli, the oxygen in the air is extracted and transferred into the bloodstream in exchange for the carbon dioxide. As you breathe in, the oxygen goes into the bloodstream and the carbon dioxide goes into the air passages. When you breathe out, you expel the carbon dioxide. The basic problem with any disease affecting the lungs is the interference with the normal exchange of oxygen for carbon dioxide.

COUGHS

What causes us to cough?

The cough reflex is a normal mechanism by which the body tries to keep the lung tissues and the bronchial trees free of any secretions or obstructions. When something irritates the lung tissue, the body responds by forcefully and involuntarily expelling air—coughing.

There are basically 2 types of coughs: a dry, nonproductive cough and a productive cough. The dry, nonproductive cough is usually caused by irritation of the cough reflex center at the back of the throat, such as that occurring with postnasal drainage, and no phlegm or material is expelled. It can also be caused by irritation from fumes, such as those from pollution or cigarette smoking.

A productive cough produces phlegm that has traveled from the lower portions of the lung and is then coughed out. Productive coughs are seen in diseases such as bronchitis, emphysema, and pneumonia.

Which cough medication is best for my cough?

The type of cough medication to use depends upon the type of cough you have and what causes that cough. If you remember, I said that there are 2 types of cough: a dry cough and a productive cough.

A dry cough is caused by irritation in the back of the throat, which can be created by postnasal drip or by inhaling fumes or toxic materials. Of course, if the latter is the case, the treatment will be to immediately get rid of the toxic materials and breathe in some warm, moist air. If, for instance, you have been exposed to the chemical chlorine, you should immediately get away from the toxic materials, go into a bathroom, shut the door, and turn the shower on scalding hot. Stay away from the water, but let the steam build up within the bathroom. Take in slow, deep breaths. That will expose the back of your throat and your lung tissue to the moisture in the steam and will help the cough created by fumes.

If, however, your dry cough is produced by an irritant in the back of the throat, such as postnasal drip, the treatment may be to take an antihistamine to reduce the postnasal drip. Many people find that once their nasal and sinus congestion is dried up, their cough quickly goes away. A cough suppressant formula with antihistamine in it is often helpful for this nagging sort of cough. Always follow the directions on the label.

If you have a productive cough, the treatment is entirely different. Since coughing is the body's way of ridding the lungs of the secretions an infection produces, a cough suppressant would reduce your body's ability to get rid of the secretions, setting up a potential situation for more infection. For a productive cough, take a cough expectorant. The expectorant in the cough medicine will help loosen the secretions in the chest, and even though this medication will not totally reduce the cough, it will cause your cough to be more productive, clearing the secretions more quickly from the lungs.

Should I be alarmed if I cough up blood?

Coughing up blood, or hemoptysis, is a warning sign of cancer. Without question, anyone who coughs up blood, especially a chronic smoker, is considered to have a serious lung problem such as cancer until it is proven otherwise. Other causes of coughing up blood include severe bronchitis; pneumonia; trauma to the breathing passages, such as swallowing or inhaling a foreign object; blood that has gotten down into the lungs from bleeding sinuses or a nosebleed. Anyone who coughs up blood should immediately contact a physician for a proper evaluation. The exact cause of that blood has to be found.

LUNG INFECTIONS

What is bronchitis?

Bronchitis is an inflammation of the bronchial tubes that can be caused by a virus or a bacterium. When either of these organisms invades the bronchial tree, an increased amount of secretions is produced that can become infected.

The symptoms of bronchitis are generally achiness, fever, and a productive cough. People with bronchitis will generally cough up phlegm that is colored brown, yellow, or green. The color of the phlegm does not reflect the seriousness of the bronchitis, unless it is red.

Most people with bronchitis will have shortness of breath because the excess secretions interfere with the normal flow of air, thus decreasing the amount of oxygen that can be taken in by the body. The diagnosis of bronchitis is usually made by evaluating the medical history and by listening to the lung fields through a stethoscope. As the physician listens for the flow of air through the lungs, loud crackling noises can be heard on both sides of the lung, indicating inflammation within the bronchial tree.

If your physician decides that your bronchitis is caused by a virus, he or she will generally prescribe a cough expectorant to help clear the secretions from your lungs and to prevent any worsening of the infection. If, however, your physician thinks that the bronchitis has been caused by a bacterial infection, antibiotics will also be added to the treatment. Most cases of bronchitis will generally clear within 4 to 5 days and should leave no permanent scarring in the lungs.

People who smoke or who have underlying problems with their lungs (such as emphysema) will generally experience more frequent cases of bronchitis and the disease will persist for a longer time when it does occur.

What is pneumonia?

Bronchitis is an inflammation of the breathing passages or bronchi, but pneumonia is an infection within the small air sacs and the lung tissue itself. Pneumonia, like bronchitis, can be caused by a virus or a bacterium, but in most cases, pneumonia is caused by a bacterial infection. Symptoms include high fever, chills, night sweats, shortness of breath, and a productive cough of infected phlegm.

Your physician can make the distinction between bronchitis and pneumonia through the use of a stethoscope. Listening to the air flow through the lungs, he or she will find sections of the lung in which air flow is not occurring since air will not flow normally through infected lung tissues. In this way, the physician can pinpoint the area of the lung in which the pneumonia is occurring. Many times, a chest x-ray will be taken to outline where pneumonia is in the lung.

If you are an otherwise healthy person, pneumonia can sometimes be treated without putting you in the hospital. Using a cough expectorant, taking appropriate antibiotics, and breathing humidified air can increase your ability to rid the lung tissue of the infection. However, an elderly person or someone with a history of lung problems will probably require hospitalization and will have to be given antibiotics intravenously (through the veins).

Is there any way to prevent pneumonia?

Although pneumonia is caused by many different types of viruses or bacteria, the most common cause is a specific bacteria—the pneumococcus. This bacteria causes pneumonia in all age groups, but especially in those who are at a high risk: people with chronic obstructive pulmonary disease; diabetics; persons living in nursing homes; and almost anyone over the age of 50.

For these people a vaccine is now available. This pneumovac significantly reduces their chances of developing pneumonia from the specific bacteria pneumococcus. I recommend that the pneumovac be given to any person suffering from a chronic illness such as lung disease, heart disease, kidney disorder, or diabetes; anyone recovering from a serious illness, especially involving the lungs; anyone currently living in a nursing home or extended care facility; and anyone over 50 years of age.

This vaccine is given approximately every 5 years, and new studies conducted by the manufacturer indicate 1 shot may last a lifetime and has very few side effects. Remember that it does not protect you from all types of pneumonia, just the kind caused by this bacteria.

CHRONIC OBSTRUCTIVE PULMONARY DISEASE

What is chronic obstructive pulmonary disease?

Chronic obstructive pulmonary disease, or COPD, includes a broad range of lung problems that fit in the basic categories of chronic bronchitis and emphysema. Chronic bronchitis is manifested by a chronic irritation in the bronchial tree while emphysema involves destruction of the air passages in the lung tissue itself. Normal air passages are very tiny, hollow branches to which balloon-shaped sacs are connected; there are literally millions within the lung tissue. But chronic irritation, multiple infections, or cigarette smoking can destroy these air sacs. With the destruction of each sac, larger cavities that do not function properly are formed. When this occurs, the exchange of carbon dioxide and oxygen is markedly reduced.

People with chronic obstructive pulmonary disease, specifically emphysema, find that the oxygen they breathe is not readily transferred into the blood. Therefore, the body suffers from a chronic lack of oxygen (hypoxia). Also, it is difficult for the body to rid itself of the waste product of carbon dioxide so that this substance builds up within the blood. The combination of the lack of oxygen within the blood system and the increased amount of carbon dioxide causes individuals with chronic obstructive pulmonary disease to suffer fatigue and a marked increase in shortness of breath with any activity.

What is chronic bronchitis?

Chronic bronchitis is a condition in which an individual has suffered repeated bouts of infections within the bronchial tree. Chronic bronchitis is a form of COPD, or chronic obstructive pulmonary disease. Individuals with chronic bronchitis generally have smoked for long periods of time or have been exposed to toxic chemicals, such as those found in industrial plants.

Chronic bronchitis can cause a person to have a chronic productive cough and to experience a decrease in lung capacity, which would manifest itself as shortness of breath. When a physician diagnoses chronic bronchitis, a primary treatment is to have the person totally avoid the offending irritants. This may include stopping smoking or removing oneself from the source of industrial pollution. The individual may also be placed on medications that will help the lungs stay as clear from secretions as possible.

It is very important for people who have chronic bronchitis to contact a doctor when any significant change occurs in their breathing patterns. People who experience an increased incidence of shortness of breath, an increase in the amount of coughing, or a change in the color of their phlegm should check with their physician.

If I have emphysema, can I make my breathing more effective?

People with emphysema often feel they always have to fight to get enough air. When they feel breathless, they become frightened and try harder to breathe. But gasping for air only makes breathing more difficult because it traps some of the stale air within the lung tissue. The best way to keep the airways open, get the stale air out, and get fresh air in is to use a breathing technique called pursed-lip breathing. Follow these steps:

1. Relax and let your neck and shoulders droop.
2. Breathe in slowly.
3. Purse your lips, as if you were whistling, and breathe out slowly and steadily—about twice as slowly as you breathe in.

Practicing pursed-lip breathing can increase the effectiveness of each breath for even the most severe chronic obstructive pulmonary disease sufferer. Many people with severe lung diseases have to use pursed-lip breathing at all times, but others can use it only when the feeling of breathlessness occurs.

If I have emphysema, will breathing exercises help?

Exercising is a very important part of your treatment if you have chronic obstructive pulmonary disease. Breathing exercises specifically allow you to make the most out of your breathing by developing a more rhythmic breathing and by slowing down your breathing rate. These exercises also increase the strength of your diaphragm muscles and make each breath more efficient.

What are some of the specific exercises that can help the chronic lung patient?

Several exercises can teach the basic techniques of breathing. If you are interested in these exercises, consult your doctor or breathing specialist about how to do them properly and about whether or not you will need to take medications before doing the exercises. Here are 2 basic, effective exercises that can help the chronic lung patient:

Exercise #1: Basic breathing

119

Lie on your back on the floor or on a firm bed. Place one hand firmly on the middle of your chest and the other on your stomach. Keeping your mouth closed, breathe in slowly through your nose and push your stomach out as far as possible. If you are breathing correctly, the hand on the stomach should move, not the one on your chest. Then purse your lips (as if you were going to whistle) and breathe out, pressing your stomach in and up toward your head. Again, the hand on your chest should not move. Practice this breathing pattern for approximately 3 minutes while lying down, and then try it again while sitting, standing, walking, and climbing stairs. Practice this form of breathing until it becomes natural.

Exercise #2: Candle blowing

Sit with your chest wall about 1′ from a table and place a candle in a candleholder on the table. Raise the candleholder so that the top of the candle is about chin height. After you light the candle, practice the basic breathing described above, blowing until the flame bends but does not go out. Practice this for approximately 3 minutes every day. On each successive day, place the candle a little farther away from you on the table. Repeat the exercise until you have increased the distance to approximately 3′ away from your chin.

These are not the only exercises you could and should do, but they are 2 basic ones that can help you. Always check with your physician as to whether these exercises can be beneficial to you and exacty how you should perform them.

Why do some people with lung disease have to be on oxygen when they are at home?

A cardinal sign of emphysema or chronic bronchitis is the inability to get enough oxygen into the bloodstream. When lung disease has progressed to the extent that the tissue has been destroyed, it may be almost impossible for an individual to get enough oxygen from breathing normal air. Many people can be helped dramatically if they can breathe a higher concentration of oxygen during certain periods of the day. These higher concentrations of oxygen are created through the use of various oxygen systems that can be used at home.

Depending upon your needs, there are 2 main types of oxygen systems. If you rarely leave home, an oxygen concentrator can supply you with an adequate amount of oxygen. The concentrator takes the oxygen from the surrounding air and delivers it to you via a tube with lightweight, hollow prongs that fit inside your nose.

If you are active and need a movable oxygen supply, a liquid oxygen system may be best. This consists of a stationary oxygen reservoir that holds 3 to 8 days of oxygen and a walker unit you can take with you. The walker unit, when full, can store approximately 8 hours of oxygen. This oxygen is also delivered through a tubing-and-prongs system.

The amount of oxygen you use each day will be prescribed by your physician, depending upon your needs. These needs will be determined by your underlying condition and the amount of oxygen you normally have in your system when you breathe room air.

Too much oxygen can be dangerous. Your doctor will determine a safe dosage, but if you exceed that dosage, you could suffer some disastrous effects.

CIGARETTE SMOKING

Can cigarette smoking cause chronic obstructive pulmonary disease?

The principal cause of chronic obstructive pulmonary disease (either chronic bronchitis or emphysema) is cigarette smoking. The repeated inhalation of smoke from cigarettes destroys not only the breathing passages, the bronchi, but also the small air sacs. Many people do not realize that the smoke inhaled from cigarettes contains tar, nicotine, and literally thousands of other potentially damaging chemicals. With every puff of a cigarette, further destruction takes place.

It is virtually assured that anyone who smokes will eventually develop some degree of chronic obstructive pulmonary disease. This generally begins in the mid- to late-40's when the individual develops a chronic cough. This cough is worse in the morning and produces a whitish phlegm. As the person gets older and the cigarette smoking continues, the coughing will worsen and be associated with a significant increase in shortness of breath and a decreased ability to exercise.

If I stop smoking, will my lung disease get better?

The only definite thing that can be said is that once you stop, your lung condition will certainly get no worse. Depending, of course, upon the amount of cigarettes you smoked and the length of time you have been smoking, the cessation of smoking will usually lead to some degree of improvement in the health of your lungs and your breathing capacity.

If a physician does a breathing test on a smoker and then repeats the test after that person has stopped smoking for 3 to 6 months, almost always some significant improvement in the breathing capacity is observed. Individuals who have COPD and stop smoking may continue to experience some coughing, but in most cases it will be significantly reduced. Chronic irritation from cigarette smoking also increases your chances of having infections within your lungs. People who stop smoking usually have a significant decrease in the number of pulmonary infections such as bronchitis and pneumonia.

Is cigarette smoking really harmful for your lungs?

Regardless of some of the propaganda that you might have read, it can definitely be stated that cigarette smoking is not only harmful but potentially deadly. Here are some facts that you should know regarding cigarette smoking and its effect upon health and, specifically, the lungs:
• Cigarette smoking is responsible for 1 in every 5 cancer deaths in our country.
• The risk of developing lung cancer is 10 times greater for cigarette smokers than nonsmokers.
• Over 346,000 deaths each year are related to cigarette smoking.
• The chance of death for an ex-smoker who has not smoked for 15 years is similar to that of someone who has never smoked.
There is no doubt that if you smoke, you have a greater likelihood of developing lung cancer and damaging your breathing passages, leading to chronic bronchitis or emphysema. Lung cancer can kill you, but these forms of chronic obstructive pulmonary disease can totally disable you.

With each breath of smoke you take, dangerous tars, nicotine, and other toxic fumes are inhaled in your breathing passages. Their effects on your breathing passages destroy not only the smaller airways but also the larger breathing passages, the bronchi. Cigarette smoking is the number 1 health hazard in this country. The vast majority of significant lung diseases could be prevented if people simply would not smoke. With all of the dangerous facts of smoking that are being relayed to the public today, it is amazing that people continue to smoke, or at least that they do not seek professional help to find effective ways to stop smoking.

ASTHMA

What is asthma?

Asthma is a disease that constricts the air passages in the lungs and causes repeated attacks of difficulty in breathing, wheezing, and sometimes coughing. The wheezing sound created during an asthma episode is much like the sound made when you blow through a straw, then gently pinch the middle of the straw.

Asthmatic attacks can occur for a variety of reasons. Some people respond to infection within the bronchial tree with a tightening sensation and wheezing. This is referred to as bronchial asthma.

Asthma can also be caused by an allergy to something within the environment. These asthma sufferers may have a sudden attack of wheezing when they are exposed to pollen in the spring. As the pollen enters the body, it causes an acute allergic reaction that produces a swelling and tightening of the air passages; the person has difficulty breathing in and expelling air. The individual will also have a feeling of suffocation, usually followed by an increase in anxiety (which further worsens the condition).

What happens during an asthmatic attack?

During an asthmatic attack, the bronchial tubes become very constricted or tight. This occurs because the muscles surrounding the bronchial tubes tighten up, leaving a much narrower airway than usual. The lining of the bronchial tubes also begins to swell, which narrows the tubes even more. Along with the swelling of the lining, an increase in the amount of mucus or secretions within the bronchial tubes occurs.

To asthma sufferers, an asthmatic attack is a sudden choking sensation—as if someone was holding a pillow tightly over the head. The person has tremendous difficulty breathing and gasps for air. A feeling of panic almost always accompanies an asthmatic attack.

The combination of these factors makes it extremely difficult to get air through the air passages. The air that is forced into the lungs by the person's gasping has an even greater difficulty getting out of the lungs, and the body struggles for oxygen with each breath.

What causes an allergic asthmatic attack?

Sometimes the asthmatic attack is triggered by an allergic reaction. This type of asthma is known as allergic asthma and generally begins in childhood. When the substance a person is allergic to—the allergen—enters the body through the air passages, the body senses it as a foreign material and begins to mobilize a force of antibodies to destroy the foreign material. When the antibodies combine with the allergen, an allergenic compound is created, which releases chemicals (histamines) that produce the asthmatic attack. The watery eyes, runny nose, skin rash, stomach upset, and other symptoms referred to as the allergy complex are all caused by the release of these histamines. The release of histamines also causes a tightening or constriction of the bronchial tubes. So, when certain allergic persons come in contact with an allergen, an acute reaction occurs, causing a constriction and tightening of the air passages—asthma.

Can asthma be triggered by things other than allergies?

In nonallergenic asthma, generally no identifiable allergen can be found that would cause an attack. This type of asthma generally does not appear until adulthood and most often follows a lung infection. There is usually no personal or family history of allergies or asthma in childhood. But, even though no identifiable substance triggers the attack, certain substances that are irritating to the person may provoke an attack. Smokers, people who are exposed to excessive amounts of dust or fumes, people who work in industrial environments full of pollution, and people with a history of respiratory infections are particularly vulnerable to this type of asthma.

How is a person with asthma treated?

Care of an asthmatic has 2 parts: emergency treatment and preventive treatment.

A person having an acute asthmatic attack is considered to be a medical emergency and must have the spasm in the bronchial tubes relieved immediately to reestablish the ability to breathe normally. In most cases, an acute asthmatic attack is treated with a medication that counteracts the allergic reaction stimulated by the chemical histamine. The most commonly used medication is epinephrine, which is given as an injection. Within 5 to 10 minutes, the epinephrine is absorbed into the blood system, and it goes immediately to the lung tissue and counteracts the constriction. Breathing can be fairly normal within several minutes.

Once the acute bronchial constriction has been treated, the physician will concentrate on the underlying cause of the asthma. For example, the physician may advise avoiding an animal that provoked the asthma attack or, if pollen is the suspected culprit, closing the windows and using air conditioning (if necessary) to keep the pollen outside. If the acute asthmatic attack has been stimulated by an infection, the physician will, of course, prescribe appropriate antibiotics.

Once the individual is over the acute episode, a maintenance program will be instituted, probably consisting of medications to counteract the allergic response and to keep the air passages open until the infection or allergic cause has been reduced or, preferably, eliminated.

What are some of the factors that can trigger an asthmatic attack?

People can be allergic to almost anything in the environment. However, through experience we know that there are some common substances that, even though they do not affect most people, can trigger an acute asthmatic attack in the allergic individual. Some of the more common ones are pollens from trees, grasses, and weeds; mold and spores; pet dander, saliva, or hair; dust; particular foods or even food aromas; certain medications; insecticides; cosmetics; and the list goes on and on.

Many nonallergenic irritants can also trigger an asthmatic attack in a susceptible individual, including the following:
• Respiratory infections
• Air pollution
• Industrial pollutants
• Tobacco smoke
• Strenuous exercise or physical exertion
• Emotional stress
• Exposure to extremes of heat or cold, dryness or humidity

A primary factor in long-term management of an asthmatic is to identify if that person is allergic to any specific substance or substances. If the individual is found to be allergic, he or she can totally avoid those irritants or perhaps be given a series of desensitization shots that build up an immunity to the asthma-causing material.

How permanent is asthma?

Asthma can occur at almost any age and it is a lifelong condition. For many people, the condition will get better as they grow older, but the possibility of a recurrent attack is still present. Unless the asthma is caused solely by an acute infection within the lungs, there is no cure. Treatment or management consists of relieving the symptoms or reducing the exposure to the asthma-causing irritants.

PLEURISY

What is pleurisy?

Each lung is surrounded by a membranous tissue called the pleura that protects the lungs within the chest cavity; the pleura is basically a sac around the lung. Pleurisy is an inflammation of this membrane.

There are basically 2 types of pleurisy, depending upon the cause. "Primary" pleurisy is an inflammation of the sac arising from a viral or bacterial infection. "Secondary" pleurisy is an inflammation of the sac created by some other condition going on within the lung tissue itself, such as pneumonia. Tuberculosis, lung abscesses, tumors of the lung, or almost any other condition within the lung tissue itself can lead to secondary pleurisy.

How can I tell if I have pleurisy?

The most common system associated with pleurisy is pain. If you go back to what the pleura is—a sac that surrounds the lung itself—you can see that any time the lung expands with normal breathing, this sac or pleura will expand, also. If the sac is inflamed or infected, then sudden expansion of the sac will cause pain. People with this condition complain of a sudden stabbing of knifelike pain directly over the area of the inflammation during deep breathing or a sudden cough or sneeze. Along with shallow, very difficult breathing and pain, other symptoms that might occur are dry coughing, weakness, headache, or loss of appetite. Chills, fever, and a rapid heart rate are not unusual. Every pain that occurs in the chest with deep breathing is not pleurisy, but when the pain is associated with fever and a cough, pleurisy becomes the most likely diagnosis.

How is pleurisy treated?

The inflammation of the pleura is best treated by curing the infection that caused it. Antibiotics will reduce infection and inflammation and thus reduce the pain. Pleurisy caused by problems within the lung tissue itself, such as pneumonia, is best treated by curing the underlying disease.

But as far as most people are concerned, the only symptom they are interested in curing is the pain. A physician can deal with the pain in a variety of ways. One way is to place the individual on pain medications, sometimes a narcotic, to reduce the pain until the underlying cause is treated. Other times the physician may elect to prescribe an anti-inflammation medicine, which will reduce the inflammation while the original infection is being cured. Applying heat to the chest wall with a heating pad or hot-water bottle can also help reduce the inflammation while the original infection is healing.

Some people think that the best way to treat pleurisy is to bind the chest in a rib-binder so that the lungs will not expand, but this can cause major difficulties, especially in elderly people. If the rib cage is bound so that the lungs do not expand properly, there will certainly be a decreased irritation of the pleura. But there will also be many deleterious effects, such as the lung tissue collapsing and setting up even more infection.

CHEST X-RAYS

How often should I get a chest x-ray to prove I don't have cancer?

If you are going to rely on a chest x-ray to find whether or not you have cancer, you're playing Russian roulette. Waiting until something shows up on your x-ray before taking serious steps toward *preventing* cancer is like closing the barn door after the horses are gone. In fact, if you get a chest x-ray and it shows a spot on the lung that could be cancer, in many cases it may be too late. You should *never* rely on a chest x-ray to decide whether or not you should stop smoking. Stop smoking now.

For people who do smoke, however, it is suggested that they have a chest x-ray every 2 to 3 years after the age of 40. This is to check on the development of any suspicious areas and the beginning stages of chronic obstructive pulmonary disease. Combined with proper breathing tests and examination of sputum, an x-ray can provide a pretty good look at the condition of the lungs.

OCCUPATIONAL HAZARDS AND THE LUNGS

How common is it for someone to develop lung problems because of their occupation?

Millions of workers in thousands of different occupations are exposed to health hazards every day because of the substances in the air they breathe on the job. It has been estimated by the American Lung Association that approximately 65,000 workers in the United States develop respiratory diseases related to their jobs and an additional 25,000 will die from occupational lung diseases.

Lung diseases can occur if the air breathed contains hazardous levels of dust, sprays, fumes, vapors, or gases. Breathing in these hazardous substances can lead to a number of lung diseases, such as chronic bronchitis, emphysema, fibrosis (a hardening of the lung tissue), and lung cancer.

What are some of the specific substances that are dangerous?

Hazardous materials take many forms. They are produced in different ways and are associated with many different types of jobs.

127

Dust. Hazardous substances in the form of dust can be found around silica, asbestos, coal, kaolin, and talc. Other dusts come from materials such as grains, coffee beans, cotton, and flax.

Fumes. Fumes are formed when solids, usually metals, are heated to extreme temperatures. The fumes that can cause lung disease come from metals such as nickel, cadmium, chromium, and beryllium. When the fumes from these metals are breathed into the lungs, their particles can cause lung inflammation, bronchitis, and lung cancer. Workers in industrial operations such as welding, smelting, furnace work, and pottery making are most often exposed.

Smoke. Smoke is formed by the burning of organic materials or from a variety of dust, gases, and vapors. Smoke inhalation, for instance, is the most common cause of injury to firefighters and can lead—if the exposure is over a long period of time—to damage to the lung tissue.

Gases. Gases are by far the most dangerous agents found in the workplace. They can suffocate a person by displacing the oxygen in the air. On the job, gases are produced by chemical reactions and high heat, such as welding, brazing, smelting, oven-drying, and furnace work. Poor ventilation and confined working areas increase the danger.

Vapors. At some point, all liquids give off a gaseous material called a vapor. In the lungs, vapor acts the same way as a gas. Vapors that can damage the lungs will usually irritate the nose and throat first, which is a valuable warning sign. Some vapors, such as water vapor, are not harmful, but others, such as solvents, can cause serious illnesses.

These are a few of the common substances that can create lung problems in the workplace. Much can be done to reduce workers' exposure to them, such as improving ventilation, training the workers to identify potential hazards, changing specific procedures that will lessen the exposure, and using protective equipment, such as respirators or special breathing masks.

8.

Heart Disease

HOW THE HEART WORKS

Why is my heart referred to as a pump?

Your body contains about 70,000 miles of blood vessels which function to carry a supply of blood to every part of your body. Your heart is the center of your circulatory system, and it pumps blood to all parts of your body. Your heart beats approximately 70 times a minute, or about 100,000 times a day, and pumps the same amount of blood throughout your circulatory system over and over again. During each heartbeat, approximately 2 to 3 ounces of blood are released to the blood vessels. The blood carries vital nutrients and oxygen that are critical to the proper functioning of your body.

Your heart is basically a simple, muscular machine—a pump. The work of the heart is done by a strong muscular wall called the myocardium. When the heart muscle tightens up, or contracts, the blood is forced out of the heart into the blood vessel system. Then the heart relaxes, allowing itself to be filled up with a fresh supply of blood. Think of how a water pump works—when the plunger is compressed, water is pushed out of the pump. When the plunger relaxes, the pump fills up with water again.

Actually, your heart has 2 pumps—1 on the right side and 1 on the left side. The function of the right pump is to receive blood that has already been utilized by your body. This blood carries within it carbon dioxide, a waste product for which your body has no use. When the right pump contracts, it squeezes the blood into the lung tissue. The blood then flows through the lungs, where the carbon dioxide is released and the vital, fresh oxygen is absorbed. This fresh blood, with its new oxygen, is then forced into the left pump and squeezed into the arteries to be delivered to all parts of your body. This cycle is repeated over 100,000 times a day, year after year.

What are heart valves?

The 2 pumps (right and left) are each composed of 2 chambers. The top chamber of each pump is the atrium; the lower chamber is the ventricle. Each chamber is separated by a door, or heart valve. When blood flows from the upper chamber, or atrium, into the lower chamber, or ventricle, the heart valve is open. When blood flows from the ventricle into the lungs or out into the circulatory system, the heart valve separating the 2 chambers closes, preventing blood from flowing back into the upper chamber. On the right side of the heart, this valve is referred to as the tricuspid valve. On the left side is the mitral valve. There are also valves separating the ventricles in each side of the heart from the lungs and the general circulation. On the right side of the heart, the valve separating the ventricle from the lungs is the semilunar valve. On the left side of the heart, the valve separating the ventricle from the general circulation is the aortic valve.

The normal heart functions in amazing synchronization so that the proper valve will shut at the proper time, allowing blood to be forced through its proper course. When a valve malfunctions, the blood flow is not maintained at a steady rate. The problem can be that the valve is too tight and fails to open properly or that the valve is too loose and simply flutters as the blood flows across it. You may have heard about someone having an aortic valve replaced. That simply means that the aortic valve separating the left ventricle from the outer circulation has malfunctioned and it had to be replaced with an artificial valve.

People with problems with the valves of the heart can suffer a variety of symptoms. Some people will have shortness of breath, because blood accumulates in the lungs and is not allowed to follow its normal course from the lungs back to the side of the heart. Other people with valve problems will suffer chest pain, because the malfunctioning valve does not allow for proper circulation through the heart's arteries.

How does my heart get its oxygen supply?

For your heart to work properly, it must have oxygen and nutrients, just like the rest of your body. A series of heart or coronary arteries situated on the outer surface of the heart supply this oxygen and nutrients. As blood leaves the left side of your heart, it begins a trip through a single major artery called the aorta, which arches over the top of your heart and passes down through your chest and into your abdomen. At the beginning of the aorta, 2 small arteries, known as the coronary arteries, branch off. They wrap around your heart muscle and divide into smaller branches, carrying the blood supply deep into every portion of your heart. The artery on the left side of your heart, the left coronary artery, divides into 2 large branches called the anterior descending branch and the circumflex branch before dividing into the smaller arteries. When doctors talk about coronary arteries in terms of 3 vessels, they are referring to the 2 main left arteries and the 1 main right artery.

The strength of your heart muscle and the length of time that it will work depend to a great extent on an adequate supply of blood being furnished through these coronary arteries. Any change in these arteries that stops or slows the flow of vital oxygen and nutrients to the heart can lead to the heart's deterioration and weakening.

HARDENING OF THE ARTERIES

What does it mean when you have hardening of the arteries of the heart?

The inside walls of the coronary arteries are normally very smooth and flexible, letting the blood flow freely. Over time, however, fats, cholesterol, and other materials carried in the bloodstream may begin to cling to the inside walls of these arteries. As this deposit, or plaque, builds up, the space inside the vessels may become narrowed or even blocked, restricting the flow of blood. This process is similar to what happens in a water pipe when rust builds up on the inside. Initially, the water will continue to flow freely because the rust is not obstructing the flow. But when the rust becomes thick and dense, as in an old iron pipe, the flow of water begins to slow down, eventually moving only in small drips or not at all. This process of the buildup of the plaque and the narrowing of the arteries is called arteriosclerosis, or hardening of the arteries.

Arteriosclerosis is a slow but progressive disease that can begin even in early childhood. Many heart specialists say that the process of arteriosclerosis begins almost at the moment of birth. However, it takes many years for the plaque to build up enough to slow down the flow of blood to the heart's arteries. In the early stages of arteriosclerosis, the blood may flow well enough to provide enough nutrients and oxygen to the heart muscle, but as the disease progresses, the time will come when the heart will not be adequately supplied. It is at this time that the heart muscle begins to be "starved" for oxygen and symptoms of hardening of the arteries of the heart begin.

How can I keep from developing hardening of the arteries of the heart?

Arteriosclerosis, or hardening of the arteries, is a natural process. Some believe it begins at birth and progresses as we get older, but in a percentage of people, it progresses at a faster rate than in others. However, there are things each of us can do to help slow this down.

There is a definite relationship between long-term high blood pressure and the development of heart disease. To lower your risk of having heart disease, it is imperative that you have your blood pressure checked frequently. If you have a family history of high blood pressure, it's even more important that your blood pressure be checked at least every 6 months. If you have hypertension or high blood pressure, then *please* follow your doctor's advice regarding its treatment. You may not be able to prevent hypertension, but you can help keep it under control. Strict adherence to diet, exercise, and medication and not smoking are essential. The payoff is that you lessen your chances of developing heart disease.

Diabetes can also lead to arteriosclerosis because it prevents the body from utilizing its sugars and, therefore, builds up sugars as starches in the blood. So, another way to guard against hardening of the arteries is to make sure that your blood sugar is normal. People over 35 who are overweight and have a family history of diabetes are particularly vulnerable.

Another preventive measure is to cut down on your consumption of alcohol. Large amounts of alcohol can damage the heart. Studies show that excessive alcohol intake can lead to high blood pressure, angina, coronary heart disease, and heart attack. Be sensible about what you drink. Understand its dangers and know your own limitations.

Regular exercise strengthens your heart and its blood vessels. A preventive measure such as a regular exercise program will ensure a stronger, healthier heart. People who exercise regularly and keep all the other factors such as blood pressure, diabetes, and cholesterol in line are much less prone to develop heart disease.

Diets high in cholesterol and fats can lead to arteriosclerosis, angina, and heart attacks. Maintaining a diet low in cholesterol and fats and keeping your weight at its ideal level are essential in the prevention of heart disease.

The number 1 health hazard in this country is smoking. Smoking constricts your blood vessels, raises your blood pressure, increases your heart rate, and increases your likelihood of having a heart attack. Smokers are 4 to 5 times more likely to develop heart disease than nonsmokers. Decreasing the number of cigarettes you smoke or better still, quitting can greatly improve your chances for a healthier future.

How can a physician tell if I have hardening of the arteries?

A physician will take a complete history and see whether or not you have any of the risk factors. He or she will also take a heart history, asking if you have any symptoms when under emotional stress or during physical exercise. If any risk factor or symptom is present, the doctor will then probably test you for high cholesterol levels and diabetes and perhaps do a heart tracing or electrocardiogram.

All these tests and questions will not necessarily provide the answer. You may have some hardening of the arteries present (as we probably all do) but not enough to cause problems. In most cases, doctors rely on the fact that if the individual is able to do normal exercise and has no risk factors present, he or she probably does not have a significant degree of hardening of the arteries. However, if you have hypertension or diabetes and if you smoke a lot you can be fairly certain that some degree of heart disease has already begun.

ANGINA

What is angina?

Angina is the common term for *angina pectoris,* which literally means "pain in the chest." Angina occurs when there is a temporary decrease in the supply of oxygen to the heart muscle. This occurs when arteriosclerosis, or hardening of the arteries, has progressed to the point of slowing the supply of blood through the heart's arteries.

To help you better understand the reasons for angina, perhaps I should explain what happens when extra demands are placed on any part of the body. Any muscle—and the heart muscle is no exception—requires a certain level of oxygen and nutrients to perform work. The more work being performed, the more oxygen is needed. Your body senses any increase in the amount of work that you are doing and tries to supply the extra needs by speeding up the heart rate and the blood supply to all parts of the body. Remember, the blood supply must be increased to carry additional amounts of oxygen. Your heart muscle functions well as long as these requirements are met.

As with any other part of the body, the requirements for oxygen and nutrients are less when the heart is at rest. As the work load is increased, the requirements are also increased. You may receive enough blood and oxygen for doing sedentary work, such as cooking or sitting at a desk job. But the moment you become more active, the supply of oxygen reaches the critical level, and you experience the muscle's reaction to a lack of oxygen—*pain.* This explains why many people with angina do all right when they are performing light tasks but experience pain when they mow the grass or walk up stairs. The heart needs more oxygen for these activities, and it cannot get it through the hardened arteries. Angina is usually characterized by a brief squeezing or tight sensation in the middle of the chest, and the pain goes away when the activity is stopped.

A typical story about someone with angina would be as follows: Mr. Smith was a 48-year-old bookkeeper. He came and went to work without any difficulty and had no idea that he might have heart problems. On a Saturday afternoon, Mr. Smith went out to mow the grass. While pushing the mower up a hill, he had a sudden squeezing sensation under his breast bone, and it frightened him. He stopped mowing immediately and sat down to rest. The pain slowly went away. He figured it was a spasm and started mowing again, but any time he tried to go up the hill, the pain returned.

From what we have just learned, we can reason that as long as Mr. Smith was mowing on level ground, his heart was getting enough oxygen, and therefore, he had no pain. But the extra work required to push the mower up the hill required more oxygen than his diseased arteries could deliver. Mr. Smith had *angina.*

If my parents had angina, will I have it?

If 1 or both of your parents have had angina or suffered a heart attack, you have an increased risk of developing that disease. This is particularly true if either of your parents suffered a heart attack before the age of 60. Some of the risk factors for heart disease tend to occur within families. Hypertension, a definite risk factor, can occur within families. Obesity, too, can occur in families because of poor dietary habits. Just because your parent had a heart attack does not automatically mean that you will. But, if either or both have had heart disease, especially before the age of 60, you should be more conscious of the risk factors of heart disease and keep your health at its optimum level.

If I have angina, does that mean I will have a heart attack?

It is not true that all people who suffer from angina will eventually have a heart attack. Many people live with the symptoms of angina for many years and are able to control these attacks through the use of proper medication. But angina is a warning sign. If your angina gets significantly worse, it could be a warning of an impending heart attack.

For example, if you have controlled the symptoms of angina by taking only 1 or 2 nitroglycerin tablets every now and then and you suddenly require 3, 4, or 5 nitroglycerin tablets a day, that is a significant indication that something is wrong. This change should be reported immediately to your physician who can then reevaluate your condition. Your physician will want to take another look at the condition of your heart and arteries to see if the circulation to your heart has been reduced to the point that you could be on the verge of having a heart attack.

If I have angina, can it be treated with medication?

After taking a complete history and doing a complete physical examination or other special testing, your physician may decide that your type of heart disease can be treated with medication. Whichever type of medication your doctor prescribes, its function will be to increase the blood flow through the coronary arteries.

There are basically 3 types of medication your physician may elect to use. The 1st is nitroglycerin, which has been prescribed for the treatment of heart disease and angina for many years. The most common form is a small nitroglycerin tablet. At the onset of chest pain or angina, a tablet of nitroglycerin is placed under the tongue, and it is rapidly absorbed through the lining of the mouth. The chemical is then transferred through the blood system to the heart where it causes an enlargement or dilation of the heart arteries. The subsequent increase in blood flow to the heart muscles will relieve the angina.

Another type of nitroglycerin, a tablet which can be taken under the tongue or swallowed, will give a longer lasting effect. Nitroglycerin can also be prescribed in the form of an ointment; a measured amount is placed on the skin, where it is absorbed slowly over a period of 2 to 4 hours. If your physician chooses to use nitroglycerin, he or she will elect 1 of the different preparations and select the correct amount and number of times per day that it should be administered. The longer acting nitroglycerin is basically used to prevent the occurrence of angina while the under-the-tongue tablets are prescribed to treat acute or sudden attacks.

A new nitroglycerin patch has also been developed. This patch containing the nitroglycerin chemical is placed on the chest wall and left for 24 hours. This way, the medication is slowly and continuously released throughout the day and night.

A 2nd type of medication used in the treatment of angina is the beta-blocker. Beta-blocker agents perform the same task as nitroglycerin by

135

increasing blood flow to the heart, but in a different way. The linings of our arteries have what are called beta-receptors. When activated, these receptors make the artery constrict. If a medication blocks this constriction, the outcome would be enlargement or dilation of the artery. Beta-blocking drugs are extremely effective in preventing, or at least reducing, the number of angina attacks. Beta-blockers are taken by mouth periodically throughout the day.

The 3rd (and relatively new) medication used to treat angina is the calcium channel blocker. Just as we have beta-receptors in our arteries, we have special mechanisms, triggered by calcium within the lining of the artery, by which the artery constricts or tightens up. If we can give a medication that will block this calcium reaction within the lining of the artery, the artery will not constrict.

If you have arteriosclerosis or hardening of the arteries and if you suffer from angina, your physician may elect to use 1 or more of these particular preparations to prevent the occurrences of angina or treat the acute or sudden attack. Make sure that you take the medication *exactly* as your physician prescribes. If you have angina, it is extremely important to keep the blood vessels of the heart open so that enough blood constantly flows to the heart muscle. Many people who once were incapacitated because of angina find that with 1 or more of these medications they can resume normal activities without having chest pain.

If I have angina, will it get worse?

Arteriosclerosis or hardening of the arteries is generally a progressive disease; you have it, and sometimes it tends to progress even further. Where once you had chest pain only with strenuous exercise, the progression of arteriosclerosis could mean that you now have chest pain with normal activities. This does not mean that everyone with angina will get worse, but it does mean that the tendency is there. If you have arteriosclerosis or angina, you must follow your doctor's advice to the letter. Not only should you take medication as prescribed, but you probably need to make significant changes in your lifestyle. If you are overweight, you need to get down to ideal body weight. If your blood pressure is elevated, you must follow your doctor's advice for getting it under control. If you have a high cholesterol level, you should get on the proper diet to bring that level down. Most important, if you smoke—*stop* smoking.

No one can guarantee that if you have angina it will not get worse. But if you control weight, blood pressure, and cholesterol level and if you don't smoke, you are in the best position to keep your angina from getting worse. If your angina does begin to worsen even with medication and changes in lifestyle, then another form of therapy could be necessary—coronary artery bypass surgery.

TESTS FOR HEART DISEASE

If I'm having chest pains, what will my doctor do to find the cause?

If a patient comes into the office complaining of chest pain, the doctor should spend a good deal of time finding out about the specifics of the chest pain. When does the pain start? What does it feel like? Where is the pain located? What happens when the patient does specific activities? The doctor will then perform a series of evaluations and tests to find if heart disease is present and, if it is, to determine its extent.

The physician will do a total physical examination to look for the presence of risk factors. An electrocardiogram or EKG will be taken to measure the electrical impulses of the heart and look for any evidence of lack of circulation.

When these tests are completed and if the physician believes that the pain comes from arteriosclerosis, additional tests may be needed to confirm the extent and severity of the problem. These tests might include a treadmill test, a thallium scan, or a cardiac catheterization to visualize the hardened arteries. These tests are safe and relatively painless and give the physician a tremendous amount of knowledge as to the extent of the heart disease.

What is a treadmill test?

Years ago, when a physician was trying to find out if a patient's heart could function properly during exercise, he would perform what is called a master's 2 step, a series of 2 steps on which the patient would rapidly walk up and down. During this exercise, the physician would constantly monitor the patient's heart. Using an EKG, the physician could watch the electrical impulse changes in the heart and determine if enough blood could get through the arteries to the heart itself.

As modern medicine has progressed, we have found more sophisticated ways to test a patient's response to exercise. Currently, the best test to evaluate a patient's response to exercise is a treadmill. In this safe, painless procedure, the patient is placed on a walking machine with wires placed on the chest to constantly monitor the heart's activity. The walking machine starts very slowly. As the test progresses, more stress is placed on the heart in a carefully controlled manner. The treadmill will go faster and the incline will increase—in other words, the patient will have to "walk" faster up a steeper "hill."

Remember that the heart may get enough blood when the heart rate is relatively slow. Under periods of increased exercise or stress, however, as the heart beats faster, it may not be able to pump enough blood through the arteries to make the muscle function normally.

During the treadmill test, the physician will constantly monitor the heart for any signs of irregularity or changes suggesting that the heart is not getting enough blood supply. If and when these irregularities show up, the test is terminated. The patient's blood pressure will also be constantly monitored to make sure that it does not rise too high during periods of stress.

All of this may sound like futuristic technology, but it is painless and extremely safe under the supervision of a qualified physician. After the test, the physician will be able to tell how your heart functions under periods of stress. If your physician has determined that the test is normal, then you probably do not have any significant narrowing of the arteries. If, however, the test has shown some degree of irritability or changes suggestive of arteriosclerosis, the doctor will advise you about the proper medical plan to significantly reduce your chances of having a heart attack.

What is a cardiac catheterization?

Cardiac catheterization is *not* surgery. It is simply a sophisticated test that a physician can use to discover any abnormalities within the heart valves, chambers, or major blood vessels or to detect the presence of fatty deposits in the coronary arteries. During the procedure of cardiac catheterization, a small tube, or catheter, is inserted into an artery or vein and passed gently through the blood vessel until it reaches the heart. Once the catheter is in position, a colorless dye is injected into the heart and moving pictures are taken of the heart's lower chambers (ventricles) and of the coronary arteries that carry the blood supply to the heart muscle.

Cardiac catheterization is a scary procedure but quite painless, and it has a minimal risk of complications. In fact, at Emory University in Atlanta, out of 100 people who undergo the test less than 1 have any problems whatsoever. According to the American Heart Association, in 1984 there were 570,000 catheterizations performed with 0.07% mortality rate.

This procedure is extremely valuable in determining exactly the condition of the coronary arteries. For some people, it may show that the chest pain they've been having is not related to fatty deposits blocking off the heart arteries. For others, it may be a lifesaving test that detects significant disease of the coronary arteries, which can then be treated.

What is an echocardiogram or "echo"?

Having an echocardiogram is similar to having a regular EKG. There is absolutely no discomfort, and it takes about 30 minutes. During an echocardiogram, you will be asked to lie flat on your back on a table. A technician will then place a small measuring device called a transducer on the left side of your chest wall. Metal plates and straps will then be placed on your arm.

The transducer sends high-frequency sound waves through the chest wall to the heart. These sound waves then bounce off certain structures within the heart and are carried back to the transducer where the sound-wave impulses are translated into an electrical impulse to be recorded on paper or on a screen.

Remember the classic World War II movies about submarines that used sonar to track ships? Sound waves sent out from the submarine would bounce off a ship or other object. The sound was recorded and then illuminated on a screen. The echocardiogram uses this same principle, except the sound waves bounce off the structures of your heart and are carried back to the transducer for illumination.

When all of the sound waves are translated into electrical impulses, these electrical impulses can be converted into a 3-dimensional picture of the inner structures of the heart. The exact size and depth of the heart chambers and the size and operation of the heart valves can be determined. Using this test, the physician can determine if a person's heart is enlarged, if the heart valves are functioning properly, or if any other abnormalities of the actual structure exist.

HEART ATTACK

What happens during a heart attack?

Blood flows through 1 of 4 main arteries in the heart to reach the heart muscle. As long as an adequate amount of blood flows through the arteries, the muscle gets the proper amount of nutrients and oxygen to function well. When the blood flow is significantly reduced, the heart muscle cannot function properly. If the blood flow is stopped entirely, the portion of the heart muscle supplied by that artery will go into severe spasms and die.

If 1 of your main heart arteries is blocked, the muscle that is supplied by that artery will then suffer ischemia, or an acute lack of oxygen. Ischemia is what causes the intense pain associated with a heart attack. If this ischemia continues for long, the heart muscle will actually die.

The portion of the heart muscle that is receiving no oxygen becomes irritable. It becomes a sort of trigger point for the rest of the heart and can suddenly begin to fire off electrical impulses. These impulses can cause the heart muscle to beat too rapidly, a condition called ventricular fibrillation. Because of this rapidness in the heartbeat, life cannot be sustained. People with this condition who do not receive immediate medical attention will die.

Now, let's assume that the artery has been blocked off and the muscle has become ischemic, but no ventricular fibrillation occurs and the patient is in a stable condition. Within 2 to 3 days after the heart attack, the body does some amazing things. It senses that the damaged heart muscle needs an increased amount of blood supply that cannot be received through the blocked artery. Therefore, the heart will actually create new arteries that move around the blocked area to the portion of the heart muscle needing the blood supply; in other words, the formation of a collateral circulation occurs. Once this circulation is complete, the damaged heart muscle receives an increased amount of blood and the extent of the damage is curtailed. This is why the period of time immediately after the heart attack is so critical—the body is waiting for that collateral circulation to form. Once it is formed, the patient is considered to be out of immediate danger and ready to begin recuperation.

A lot of people ask how a physician knows if a patient has truly had a heart attack. Of course, the pain the patient suffers helps the physician in this determination. But there are some important tests the physician will perform during the patient's 1st 3 to 4 days in the hospital. Heart muscle that has been damaged releases certain chemicals into the blood system. These chemicals, called heart enzymes, can be tested through the blood and can indicate the extent of damage to the muscle. When your physician talks about having to get back the results of your blood tests, he is actually looking for evidence in the blood of the damaged heart muscle. Angina, which is simply a decrease in the blood supply, will not cause actual damage or an elevation in the heart enzymes, but a heart attack will dramatically increase the level of heart enzymes in the blood.

Another way the physician will be able to tell whether or not you have suffered an acute heart attack is by looking at your heart tracing or electrocardiogram. When the heart muscle is damaged, it cannot carry electrical impulses through the heart. Because the electrocardiogram tests the electrical impulses, any irregularities or abnormalities indicate zones of dead or damaged heart muscle. As your physician reads your cardiogram, he or she is looking for patterns in the heart tracing that indicate damage. The combination of classic pain, elevated heart blood enzymes, and characteristic changes in the heart tracing can all lead to the definite diagnosis that a heart attack has occurred and damaged heart muscle has resulted.

Why do some people who suffer a heart attack die immediately?

The American Heart Association estimates that about 50% of the people who have acute heart attacks die before they reach the hospital. The reason for this is an acute irregularity in the heartbeat. During the heart attack, when the blood supply has been cut off to a portion of the heart, the heart becomes extremely irritable. Instead of beating normally, it begins to beat very rapidly, almost as fast as the fluttering of a butterfly's wings. Instead of beating 72 times a minute, the heart rate rises to about 350 times a minute. When this happens, the heart cannot fill with blood or pump blood to the other portions of the body—it is beating, but not really working. As noted before, this is ventricular fibrillation. People who die suddenly from an acute heart attack die not necessarily from the heart attack but from ventricular fibrillation.

How is an acute heart attack treated?

A person who suffers symptoms that point to an acute heart attack must get help immediately. In an emergency room, the heart can be constantly monitored, and if an episode of ventricular fibrillation occurs, medications and procedures can be used to control the fluttering heart. The individual's heart should be constantly monitored for any other signs of irregularities or complications. After becoming stable, a person who has had an acute heart attack is placed in a special monitoring unit, the coronary care unit, where intensive medical and nursing care can be given. The coronary care unit is a great advance in the treatment of heart attack patients and is the reason why not as many people die from heart attacks today as 10 to 20 years ago.

When any part of the body is damaged, it repairs itself much better if it is given rest. When someone breaks a bone, it will repair itself when a cast is applied so that the bone is protected and not overutilized. Of course, we can't put the heart in a cast, but we can help it to heal itself, using bed rest for the 1st 2 to 4 days after a heart attack.

The critical period after a heart attack is generally the 1st 2 to 7 days. This is the time when complications such as congestive heart failure, ventricular fibrillation, or other irregularities could arise and cause a worsening of the original heart attack or death. Because of the constant monitoring that takes place in the coronary care unit, these potentially life-threatening complications can be detected early and treated.

141

Coronary care units, however, cannot work miracles. If someone has a major heart disease and the heart muscles have deteriorated over a period of time, even today's advancements in medical technology may be unable to help.

If you have a heart attack, are you an invalid for the rest of your life?

As recently as 20 or 30 years ago, this may have been true, and many people today still believe if you've had a heart attack, "normal" life is over. This, of course, is not the case because most people are not only normal, they're often better than they used to be. It's too bad that it takes a heart attack to motivate many people to change some of their unhealthy lifestyles. People who have had heart attacks must pay more attention to the risk factors of heart disease and work toward reducing these factors. Smokers who have heart attacks need to quit smoking. Those who are overweight or have high blood pressure or high cholesterol levels, need to lose weight, lower their blood pressure, and get the fat out of their diets. A normal lifestyle after a heart attack means a better, healthier lifestyle.

This lifestyle doesn't have to be boring. In fact, I know many people who, after a heart attack, lead even better lives. Recently I treated a 42-year-old male patient who smoked a great deal, was overweight, and did not exercise. But the dramatic impact of having a heart attack motivated him to change his poor lifestyle patterns. He gave up smoking, lost weight, and began a supervised exercise program. A year after his heart attack, he was certainly not an invalid. In fact, he told me that he had never been in better health—he was happier and healthier and leading a more productive life than ever before.

What happens after a person leaves the coronary care unit?

Years ago, doctors believed that patients who had had a heart attack required bed rest for 2 or 3 weeks. However, studies over the past several years have shown that with an uncomplicated heart attack, it is much more important to get the patient started on a specific program that gradually increases the amount of exercise. In this particular program, the coronary rehabilitation program or CRP, patients who have suffered an acute heart attack are placed on a gradually increasing exercise program in a special unit within the hospital. With the care of experienced staff and constant monitoring of the heart, patients start a carefully supervised, step-by-step program of exercise. The 1st step may be exercising in bed—just moving the arms and legs. As the patient is able, the program will be gradually increased so that he or she does more active exercise while still in bed. After 4 or 5 days, the patient will get out of bed and, again under supervision be allowed to do some specific exercises. About 6 to 7 days after the acute heart attack, the patient will get up and be allowed to walk, gradually increasing the length of exercise. After 10 days to 2 weeks, the patient will be up, walking in the hall, for increasing distances and time, gradually increasing the stress on the heart. This coronary rehabilitation program has been tremendously beneficial in the recuperation of acute heart attack patients.

How soon can I get back to work after I have an acute heart attack?

It depends upon the seriousness of your heart disease, the amount of damage that was done at the time of your heart attack, and the kind of work you do. Most people with uncomplicated heart attacks can expect to get back to work at least part-time within 2 to 3 months. With the advances in heart medications and rehabilitation programs, most people lead fairly normal lives within a very short period of time.

Can I return to a normal sex life if I've had a heart attack?

Sexual activity causes the heart to beat faster, and some people with heart disease suffer from angina during intercourse. That can place a lot of emotional strain on a marriage. Sometimes even the *fear* of having the chest pain can interfere with a normal sex life. In most cases, there is absolutely no reason why the couple can't return to a normal sex life within a reasonable period of time. You may have suffered a good deal of your chest pain during intercourse before the heart attack, but with proper medication and precautions, that pain can be treated now and you can return to normal sexual activities without chest discomfort or angina. If this is a concern for you, please discuss it openly and honestly with your physician. That can save a lot of emotional anguish later on. Many times a wife will come to me and say she'd rather just avoid the sexual activity rather than risk having her husband do any more serious damage to his heart. Again, this is not the case in the vast majority of patients. Many times doctors will suggest that patients take some of the nitroglycerin preparations before having sexual intercourse. This can relieve or prevent the chest pain.

If a portion of my heart has been damaged, will it ever become normal again?

When a section of your heart muscle has been damaged because of a heart attack, the healing process begins immediately. This process, collateral circulation, takes place through the formation of new blood vessels on about the 4th day after your heart attack. These new vessels reach around the blocked areas of the normal artery and resume the blood supply to oxygen-starved tissue. The other normal arteries of the heart will also try to pick up some of the load by increasing their circulation to the heart muscle. Depending upon the amount of damage that has been done, it usually takes anywhere from 4 to 6 weeks for the heart to form enough collateral circulation to repair the injury.

If the heart damage has not been too extensive, and the collateral circulation is good, there's a chance that the heart muscle can be revived without forming a scar. If this occurs, even though you have suffered a significant heart attack, no damaged area will remain.

However, sometimes the damage is so significant that the damaged area cannot be totally repaired. If this happens, scar tissue begins to form about the 3rd week after the injury. Scar tissue is the body's response when the damage is so great that the cells cannot replace themselves. If scar tissue forms in that section of the heart muscle, the muscle will never function properly and will remain dead for the rest of your life.

If I've had 1 heart attack, will I have another?

The answer to this question depends on the extent of your underlying heart disease. Some people have only 1 of their heart arteries involved with the disease. After an acute heart attack, when collateral circulation is restored, they have no more chest pain. And if they maintain a healthier lifestyle by controlling hypertension, stopping smoking, eating a low-cholesterol diet, and exercising, the chances are relatively good that they will not have any further problems with angina or heart attacks.

However, if the individual's underlying disease involves all of the heart arteries, even if only 1 of those arteries blocks off during an acute heart attack, there is always a chance that, in the future, 1 of the other arteries may become blocked or diseased and cause another heart attack. That's why it's so important for people with heart disease to be totally evaluated to determine the extent of their disease. If a heart attack patient is found to have blockage in the other arteries, surgery may be recommended to prevent the occurrence of a heart attack in the future.

Giving patients some of the newer heart medications may significantly reduce their chances of the recurrence of heart attacks. With a combination of current medications, rehabilitation programs, and proper follow-up, your chances of future problems with your heart are significantly reduced. Once you have had a heart attack, however, it does mean that you and your physician need to work together, in a lifelong commitment, to keep you in good health.

SURGICAL AND NONSURGICAL PROCEDURES

Can surgery help a person with hardening of the arteries?

The major problem with hardening of the arteries of the heart is that the blood cannot get through the narrowed artery (or arteries). When this narrowing or blockage becomes so severe that medication is of no help, coronary bypass surgery may be recommended.

The whole purpose of the surgery is not to repair the damaged artery but to go around it. During this procedure, a long, or saphenous, vein is taken from your leg. (Don't worry, you can lose that vein without any problems in your leg.) The surgeon will open up your chest wall and expose your heart. When this is done, he or she will take the vein from your leg and sew 1 end of it to the large artery (aorta) as it leaves the heart. A channel will be created from the aorta into that end of the vein. The other end of the vein is sewn into the diseased artery, past the area of blockage. Blood can then flow from the aorta through the vein into the normal artery beyond the blockage and thus increase the blood supply to the heart muscles.

Coronary bypass surgery is different in everyone. Some people need only 1 artery bypassed, while others will have 2 or 3 blocked arteries and require double or triple bypass surgery.

Is coronary bypass surgery dangerous?

Any surgery on the heart has to be considered dangerous. However, because of advances in the technique and the skill of surgeons, the American College of Cardiology reports that the number of people who die from complications of the surgery is less than 2 in 100. This is a significantly low rate and is significantly lower than several years ago. A large number of people who require this surgery certainly could not live without it. Of course, the complications from this bypass surgery depend on a person's age and the extent of heart disease present prior to surgery. Actual risk should always be discussed with your doctor.

Of course, the danger and complications from the surgery are directly related to the extent of damage present before the surgery is done. For some people, circulation has been good enough to maintain a relatively healthy muscle, despite the artery disease. For others, the angina has been severe enough and the blood supply reduced to the extent that over a period of years the heart muscle has become very weak from lack of oxygen. Obviously, when more than 1 artery is involved and the more diseased or weakened the heart muscle has become, the more serious the surgery.

Will coronary bypass surgery cure my disease?

Coronary bypass surgery will not cure your heart disease; what it does is bypass a diseased artery, allowing increased blood flow to the heart muscle. In 80% to 90% of the cases, this surgery will significantly reduce the symptoms of pain associated with coronary arteriosclerosis.

However, for people who are severely incapacitated because of angina, this surgery can allow them to lead a more healthy, active life and can decrease their chances of having a heart attack in the near future.

The decision to have coronary bypass surgery is, of course, very serious. Make sure that when a doctor has recommended the procedure for you that you are absolutely sure exactly why the surgery has been recommended and what benefits you can expect to derive from it. If there is any doubt in your mind as to whether or not you should undergo this surgery, go to another doctor and get a 2nd opinion.

If an artery in my heart has been blocked by a blood clot, can that clot be dissolved?

A medication is now available that can potentially dissolve a blood clot lodged in an artery of the heart. This medication, streptokinase, is injected through a catheter in the vein; then it travels to the heart and works to dissolve a clot that blocks a major artery. Streptokinase treatment is not effective for everyone, but studies show that this therapy can reduce the size of the clot so that enough blood can get to the muscle of the heart and keep it from being severely damaged.

What is angioplasty?

If an individual is found to have isolated blockage of 1 of the arteries of the heart, it may be possible for this blockage to be significantly reduced without surgery. A marvelous advance that has taken place in the treatment of heart disease has been the development of a procedure called angioplasty, or balloon procedure. During this procedure, a small catheter or tube is threaded through the body into the affected artery to the point where the blockage occurs. When the catheter is passed into the middle of the blockage, a balloon located at the tip of the catheter is blown up, enlarging and improving the area.

A patient of mine complained of chest pains while playing tennis. He was given a coronary arteriogram, which showed significant narrowing of only a portion of a major heart artery. The next day, the patient had the catheter inserted and threaded to the area where the blockage occurred. The balloon was blown up and the blockage was compressed outward, significantly improving the blood flow through the portion of the artery. This patient was able, a week later, to play 3 sets of tennis without any pain.

Of course, angioplasty is not beneficial for everyone, but in selected cases, it is a significant noninvasive procedure for the improvement of heart disease. Noninvasive means the patient does not undergo an operation, which means less pain and a shorter recuperation period. Angioplasty is an advance in the treatment of heart disease that significantly improves the prognosis of patients with very isolated narrowing of the coronary arteries.

HEART FAILURE

My mother has told me that she had heart failure. I didn't realize that the heart could fail.

The heart is probably one of the most durable parts of the body, beating over the course of a normal life an estimated 3 billion times. Over the years, however, this constant work can produce some wear and tear within the heart muscle. Heart failure, also called "heart dropsy" or congestive heart failure, is usually caused by some underlying disease such as hardening of the arteries of the heart or arteriosclerosis. If the heart muscle has not received enough blood over a long period of time, the muscle will weaken and not beat effectively.

A common symptom of heart failure is increasing shortness of breath, especially when you do any kind of work, when you exercise, or when you lie down at night. This shortness of breath can also be accompanied by swelling in the ankles and by palpitations. All of these symptoms occur because the heart is not pumping the blood as effectively as it once did. Fluids will pool in the lungs, interfering with the normal exchange of oxygen. Because the normal action of the heart keeps fluids from accumulating in the legs, a heart that has "failed" will simply not be able to clear the fluids, and thus the ankle swelling occurs.

There are other causes of heart failure such as high blood pressure, alcoholism, infectious diseases of the heart muscles, and failure of a heart valve.

Most people with heart failure can be treated. However, if the arteries to the heart have been severely diseased for long periods of time or if there are other underlying problems such as a lifelong exposure to alcohol, sometimes even the best medications cannot help.

147

Can congestive heart failure be treated?

As with most other problems of the heart, the earlier the diagnosis of congestive heart failure is made, the more likely physicians are to be able to help. The heart is suffering from weakness, and a principal treatment is to give a medication called digitalis (such as Lanoxin). The digitalis helps strengthen the muscle fibers and causes the heart to beat more effectively.

Diuretics are also given to help rid the body of the excess fluid load. The less fluid there is in the system, the easier it will be for even the slightly diseased heart to pump effectively.

DIURETICS

Are all diuretics the same?

Several different types of diuretic medications are available. There is 1 specific type that rids the body of excess salt and water and, unfortunately, also causes the body to lose potassium, an element critical to the proper functioning of the heart. When a diuretic is prescribed, your doctor will probably also put you on potassium tablets or liquids. If you take potassium, follow your doctor's directions closely, *never* stop the potassium, and have the level of potassium in your blood checked regularly.

The advantage of the potassium-sparing diuretics such as aldactone or triamterene is that they can, in some people, cause a reduction in excess fluid without lowering the body's potassium level. However, such diuretics are not effective in certain people, and your doctor might prefer giving you a stronger medication with the potassium supplement.

Regardless of the type of diuretic you use, ask your doctor if you should increase the amount of potassium in your diet. Drinking orange juice and eating bananas are 2 good ways to get more potassium.

People who have had heart failure should also significantly reduce their salt intake. The more salt taken in, the more fluids retained, and the more fluids retained the more problems a heart can have.

HIGH BLOOD PRESSURE AND EXERCISE

If I've been told I have high blood pressure, does that mean I cannot exercise?

Absolutely not. Unless there is significant heart disease or another medical problem, people with high blood pressure not only can but should exercise. In fact, in the beginning treatment of high blood pressure, the physician may recommend that the patient lose weight, reduce salt intake, and begin a regular exercise program.

You are to be cautioned, however, that if you are over 40 years of age, have a family history of heart disease, are more than 15 to 20 pounds overweight, or have other medical problems, you should *never* begin an exercise program until you have checked with your physician. If your physician clears you, an appropriate exercise plan can be recommended to fit your age and medical problems.

EDEMA (SWELLING)

I have a lot of swelling in my legs. Does this mean that I have a serious problem?

An abnormal accumulation of fluid in any part of the body is referred to as edema. Because we are erect animals, this edema will usually show up as swelling of the lower legs or ankles. Edema is not a disease in itself; it is a symptom that something else is wrong. To be able to effectively treat the edema, the physician must find the underlying causes.

In young women, the most common cause of edema is too much salt in the diet. Reducing salt intake by not shaking salt at the table and avoiding salty foods (remember to read the labels) can help a great deal.

Another cause of edema is a malfunctioning of the veins in the lower legs which cannot clear the fluid out of the legs. If you have varicose veins or a blockage of a vein in your leg, you can develop swelling of the feet and ankles. This occurs most commonly in people who have a job that requires a lot of standing.

Swollen ankles or "edema" can also be caused by wearing tight garters, rolled stockings, or other constricting garments. In these instances, simply taking off the constriction will relieve the swelling.

However, edema can also be an indication of the beginnings of problems with kidney, liver, or heart. A frequent cause of edema is congestive heart failure, a condition in which the heart fails to pump effectively. Kidney and liver disorders are also common causes of edema. If your kidneys are not functioning well enough, they cannot excrete or eliminate the appropriate amount of salt. The salt will, therefore, build up within the system and cause a retention of fluid, which can lead to edema.

If you are having repeated episodes of swelling, especially if it involves both legs and especially if it is associated with any shortness of breath, you should check with your physician.

If I find some swelling in my legs, can I take an over-the-counter diuretic?

No. Edema is a sign that something is going wrong in the body, and it should never be treated as a problem in itself. The cause of your edema should always be ascertained by your physician. If a simple cause is found, a diuretic may be prescribed, which will help rid your body of the excess fluid.

Many people who take over-the-counter diuretic medications without their physician's approval can get into serious problems. Taking these medications could lead to losing too much fluid, a depletion of the body's salt and potassium levels, and a feeling of weakness and muscle cramps. Never take diuretics without consulting your physician.

IRREGULAR HEART RATE

What are palpitations?

Many people will complain that occasionally their heart races away, pounds rapidly, skips a beat, or feels as if it "flip flops." All of these symptoms are grouped into a category referred to as palpitations. Technically, palpitations simply mean rapid or irregular beating of the heart.

Palpitations can be caused by many problems. Many times a sensation of palpitations occurs under periods of stress. In otherwise healthy people, this is a fairly normal finding, and the sensation will generally go away when the episode of stress is over. Palpitations may also indicate a rapid heart rate, sometimes as much as 120 to 150 times a minute (the normal heart rate is 70 to 80 beats a minute). If you notice that at certain times your heart begins to "palpitate" and beat rapidly and then suddenly returns to normal, you could be suffering from a condition known as PAT, paroxysmal atrial tachycardia. PAT is a common finding in otherwise healthy people, especially in young women. Although it is not a dangerous heart problem, it may require medications prescribed by your physician.

Palpitations associated with shortness of breath or chest pains can also be signs of underlying heart problems, such as hardening of the arteries or congestive heart failure. Any symptoms of palpitations that occur frequently and without obvious reasons should be reported to your physician for proper evaluation.

Once it has been determined that there are no underlying problems with your heart or circulatory system, you may simply be reassured and asked to live with the problem. Lifesyle changes, such as cutting down on your daily intake of caffeine and stopping smoking, can help reduce palpitations in many people.

150

My doctor has said that I might need a pacemaker. What is a pacemaker, and why would I need it?

Your heartbeat is controlled by an electrical charge that spreads from certain points within the heart and causes your heart muscle to squeeze or contract. When this electrical activity is altered, problems can arise. Problems with this electrical circuitry can cause the heart rate to slow down, a condition referred to as bradycardia. If the heart rate slows too much, the heart is not able to pump enough times to get an adequate supply of blood to the brain and other vital organs.

A slow heart rate, or bradycardia, can be caused by many conditions. In the elderly, it can be caused by a lack of sufficient blood supply to these electrical trigger points, which can cause a very slow heart rate. This slow pulse rate can cause episodes of fainting and a lack of energy.

When the heart rate has slowed to the point that the person is beginning to get symptoms from bradycardia, it may be necessary to provide an extra booster to the electrical impulse. This can be accomplished through the insertion of a pacemaker, which is a small wire passed through a vein and embedded in the heart muscle. The wire is then attached to a battery that produces an electrical charge. This electrical charge is set at a certain rate to stimulate the heart, which will be the new rate at which the heart beats. For instance, if your heart has slowed to 40 or 50 beats a minute, a pacemaker could be inserted to increase your heart rate to around 70.

A less common reason to insert a pacemaker is when the heart rate becomes too erratic, that is, you are having a lot of extra heartbeats (an ectopic rhythm). When these extra beats come from the lower chamber or ventricle, they are referred to as PVC's, or premature ventricular contractions. When these get out of hand and cannot be controlled with medications, the condition can be very serious. This is a rare occurrence, but the insertion of a pacemaker can control the heart rate and thus the irregularity of the heart.

What causes my heart to skip a beat?

The normal rhythm of your heart is controlled by an electrical pathway. A triggering point, the SA (sinoatrial) node, fires off and sends an electrical charge throughout the upper chamber of the heart. The electrical charge then passes through another trigger point, the AV (atrioventricular) node, and sends the charge throughout the lower chamber. As the electrical impulse travels in a smooth fashion along the normal pathway, the heart contracts, thus creating your heartbeat.

For many reasons, this electrical pathway can be interrupted. When this occurs, the heart may beat irregularly. Also, there can be areas within the heart that will "fire off" spontaneously and create a skipped beat.

Almost all of us will at some time skip a heartbeat. You will feel as if your heart suddenly pounds hard and then pauses for a second before it beats again. In normal healthy people, this usually does not indicate severe heart disease and can be brought on by exercise, anxiety, too much caffeine, or no reason at all.

However, in people over the age of 40 and in people with known heart disease, this experience can indicate that an area in the lower chamber of the heart, the ventricle, is not receiving enough blood supply through diseased arteries and thus has become irritable. That irritable point can occasionally fire off by itself causing an extra beat, referred to as a PVC (premature ventricular contraction). If this happens to you, you need a thorough evaluation by your physician. Your physician will want to make sure that these PVC's are not an indication of previously undiagnosed hardening of the arteries of the heart.

PVC's in healthy people do not need to be treated. When their cause is understood, patients generally tolerate them very well. However, because of the potential in older people for these PVC's to fire off too rapidly and interfere with the normal functioning of the heart, most physicians will place them on medications to suppress or neutralize the effect of the irritated point in the ventricle.

MITRAL VALVE PROLAPSE

What does it mean when someone has a floppy heart valve?

Harvard Medical School reports that mitral valve prolapse, also called floppy heart valve or Barlow's syndrome, is found in 5% to 10% of otherwise healthy people, but it is much more common in young women between the ages of 20 and 40 and in young athletes.

The heart is normally divided into 4 chambers. The 2 chambers on the left are separated by a heart valve called the mitral valve. Normally, this valve opens and shuts with a very smooth action, but for some still-unknown reason, in people with mitral valve prolapse the valve shuts with a floppy motion. As a result, a special heart sound or murmur or a clicking sound can be heard. In fact, the whole condition has been referred to as the click-murmur syndrome.

Although this is not a serious heart condition and does not mean that you have "a bad heart," there are some symptoms that can be created in people with mitral valve prolapse. Many people, for instance, will experience some fatigue, palpitations, occasional spells of passing out, chest pains, and a feeling of nervous tension or anxiety. The reason people have these symptoms with mitral valve prolapse is not entirely understood. However, it is probably the most common reason for people in the younger age group to experience a sensation of skipped beats or palpitations.

If mitral valve prolapse is found, again it does not mean that you have a bad heart or serious heart disease. It might mean, however, that your palpitations or other symptoms could be helped by placing you on a medication referred to as a beta-blocker. Beta-blockers such as propranolol have been found to help the symptoms of mitral valve prolapse.

The only precaution necessary for people with mitral valve prolapse is the taking of antibiotics before major surgical or dental procedures. The antibiotics will help protect this floppy valve from becoming infected. Otherwise, people with mitral valve prolapse can lead normal, active lives.

9.

Problems with the Circulation

LEG PAIN

What causes the pain I get in my legs when I walk too much?

Pain in the legs (especially the calves), created by walking great distances and relieved by rest, is referred to as claudication. When this pain occurs every now and then, it is referred to as intermittent claudication.

The muscles, like any other part of the body, need a certain amount of oxygen and nutrients to work properly. When muscles are exercised, they require more oxygen and nutrients than when at rest. In certain people, especially the elderly, the arteries that supply the muscles in the back of the leg can become diseased and thickened with a plaque formation similar to what forms in the arteries of the heart—atherosclerosis. At rest, the muscles get enough blood through those diseased arteries, but when an extra demand is placed on them through exercise, the muscles suffer from a lack of oxygen and nutrients and thus cramp up. This is almost like the process of angina that occurs in the heart muscles. This "angina of the leg muscles" is created by vascular problems in the leg.

If I have "angina of the leg muscles," how can it be treated?

If you are having angina of the legs, you should see your physician who will evaluate the circulation in your legs. If the circulation is bad, a vascular flow study will probably be used to evaluate the extent of the disease. In this test, your circulation is evaluated through the use of a special machine that checks the intensity of the pulse in the major ar-

154

teries of the legs. This is checked when you are at rest and checked again after you have been exercising in the laboratory.

Many people with severe claudication have to be treated surgically. The blocked arteries leading to the muscles of the legs have to be removed and replaced with synthetic arteries or "cleaned out" to remove the plaque formation.

Your physician might also recommend the use of medication to increase the amount of blood getting through the arteries. This controversial approach is ineffective in many patients, but it might be worth a try.

There are, however, some self-help recommendations for people whose disease is not extensive. Daily exercise is tremendously beneficial because it increases the blood flow to the lower legs and strengthens the muscles. Dr. Jay D. Coffman of Boston University School of Medicine reports approximately 75% to 90% of people who have claudication are smokers. Smoking is bad for your circulation and, therefore, should be stopped. Obese people have a great deal of trouble with claudication because of their weight. A weight-reduction program with special emphasis on reducing the amount of cholesterol (which can cause plaque formation) is important. Some conditions associated with increased claudication, such as diabetes, hypertension, and high cholesterol, must be looked for and corrected.

I don't have pain in my calves when I walk too much, but they do cramp at night. What can cause this?

Nocturnal leg cramps are very debilitating. A typical sufferer goes to bed feeling fine only to awaken in the middle of the night with severe cramping in the legs. It feels as if the leg muscles have been tied up in knots. Most people will have to jump out of bed and walk around to work the tightness out before they can go back to sleep.

In the vast majority of cases, physicians don't know exactly why people have these severe nighttime leg cramps. We do know, however, that low potassium and low calcium can add to the problem. But if both of these are normal in your blood system, you fall in the category of the unknown causals.

There are several ways these nighttime leg cramps can be treated. Many people get a significant amount of relief by performing certain exercises before they go to bed. For example, you can try standing close to a wall and placing your hands on it, getting up on your toes and back on your heels, stretching your calf muscles for approximately 5 minutes before you retire.

Because we do not know exactly why most people experience leg cramps, the treatment is very difficult. Certain medications can be taken before going to bed to decrease their frequency. If you are suffering from nocturnal leg cramps, consult your physician. You may benefit from either exercise or medication.

COLD HANDS AND FEET

My hands and feet always seem to be cold. Does this mean that I have circulation problems?

The majority who suffer from cold hands and cold feet do not have circulation problems. In fact, a check on their circulation usually indicates that they have good, strong pulses carrying an adequate amount of blood to the hands and feet.

However, people with the unusual problem known as Raynaud's phenomenon experience an acute sensitivity of the very small arteries in the hands and feet that causes these small arteries to occasionally clamp off and create a feeling of coldness. The characteristic of Raynaud's phenomenon is that, on exposure to cold, the fingers will blanch white (when the blood vessels clamp off) and then turn beefy red (created by a sudden dilation or widening of the small arteries flooding the extremity with blood).

People with Raynaud's phenomenon should be checked by a physician because an underlying disease may be causing it. Raynaud's disease is a specific disease that causes these symptoms, and it occurs in lupus, rheumatoid arthritis, and other circulatory problems. Raynaud's phenomenon is also more common in smokers than in nonsmokers.

There is no specific treatment for this problem except to make sure that, on exposure to the cold, these people wear gloves and extra stockings. For instance, some people who suffer from Raynaud's phenomenon have to wear gloves when they put something in or take something out of the freezer. Just this short exposure can create the problem. Also, it is extremely important for smokers to stop smoking.

PHLEBITIS

What is phlebitis and how is it treated?

Phlebitis is an inflammation of a vein, most commonly a vein of the leg. Because of overuse, prolonged standing, and preexisting varicose veins, these veins can become irritated, inflamed, and swollen.

In the leg are really 2 different venous systems; closer to the surface of the skin are the superficial veins and deeper in the muscles lies the deep vein system. Either system can become inflamed, but the seriousness and the treatment are different for each.

Superficial phlebitis generally causes redness, warmth, and tenderness of the affected vein. It is best treated with rest, elevation of the leg, warm compresses, and occasionally aspirin. It will usually go away in 2 to 3 days.

However, inflammation of the deep vein system is an entirely different problem. When the veins lying deep in the leg become inflamed, they can also become congested with blood and form a thrombus, or clot. This condition is known as thrombophlebitis and, in addition to the above causes, can occur because of prolonged bed rest, pregnancy, the use of high-estrogen birth control pills, congestive heart failure, or obesity.

Thrombophlebitis is a serious condition because when the clot forms and becomes inflamed, it can potentially break loose and travel through the blood system to vital organs such as the lungs (a pulmonary embolus). If this occurs, the person's life is at risk, and special medical treatments must be started immediately. These patients are generally treated within the hospital with strict bed rest and the use of a blood-thinning medication, heparin, given through the veins. Depending upon the extent of the clot and inflammation, this treatment may have to be carried on for 5 to 7 days. Generally after the swelling, redness, and tenderness have gone away, the patients will be changed to a blood-thinning medication, Coumadin, that can be given by mouth. This will be continued for several months to prevent clot reformation. Coumadin is generally safe when taken under the direction of a physician, but patients should be cautious about bleeding from cuts or tooth extractions while taking a blood thinner. Also *do not* take any other medication while taking Coumadin without checking with your physician first.

10.

High Blood Pressure

BLOOD PRESSURE

What is blood pressure?

Your heart and your blood vessels make up your body's distribution, or circulatory, system. Your life depends upon this system because the blood carried throughout the body carries the vital food and oxygen supply necessary for normal functioning.

Your heart functions as the center for this circulatory system and is the pump that pushes the blood through all of the blood vessels. When your heart beats, blood is forced through the arteries of the body and a certain pressure, your blood pressure, is maintained in them. Another way to look at blood pressure is that your heart creates, or generates, the pressure and your arteries hold the pressure.

SYSTOLIC AND DIASTOLIC PRESSURE

How is blood pressure measured?

Blood pressure is measured by a *sphygmomanometer*—a Greek word meaning "pulse measurement." The sphygmomanometer or blood pressure cuff is an inflatable cuff that is wrapped around your arm above the elbow. A tube connects this cuff to a measuring device that contains a column of mercury. The cuff is inflated until the main artery located under the cuff is squeezed tightly enough to shut off the blood flow. The physician or nurse then places a stethoscope over the artery and slowly deflates the cuff. As the pressure against the artery is reduced, the physician notes when the sound of the artery can 1st be heard. This sound is the maximum pressure that is maintained within your system when the heart is contracting—your systolic pressure. As the cuff continues to deflate, another reading is recorded when the pulse sound disappears. This is the minimal pressure maintained in the arteries between the heartbeats—your diastolic pressure.

Typically, your blood pressure reading will have 2 numbers, for example, 120 over 80. The upper number is the systolic blood pressure, and the lower number is the diastolic blood pressure. A person with a blood pressure reading of 120 over 80 maintains a pressure of 120 each time the heart beats and a pressure of 80 when the heart is at rest.

How can you know if your blood pressure is too high?

Blood pressure is not a constant measurement; it does not stay exactly the same 24 hours a day, 7 days a week. Your blood pressure will fluctuate somewhat throughout the day depending upon your level of activity, the amount of coffee you drink, the amount of stress you are under, or the amount of exercise you get. It is not uncommon for someone who has a blood pressure of 140 over 80 in the early morning to have a reading of 145 over 84 late in the afternoon. This does not mean that the person's blood pressure has gotten high; it simply is the normal variation seen in almost everyone's blood pressure.

How do we determine whether or not a person has high blood pressure? A reading of 140 over 90 is the maximum blood pressure acceptable in most people. If your blood pressure averages above a systolic pressure of 140 or a diastolic pressure of 90, then you have high blood pressure. The diastolic pressure is the most critical measurement; it is used to gauge high blood pressure in most people.

If someone's blood pressure is taken and it is 145 over 94 a physician does not immediately make the diagnosis of high blood pressure. The key word is *average*—a person's blood pressure should be checked 3 to 4 times over a period of two weeks to make sure that it is *averaging* above the level of 140 over 90. Someone who goes out and wrecks the car may well have blood pressure of 150 over 95, but that doesn't mean the person has high blood pressure. The excitement of the automobile accident caused the blood pressure to be elevated at that time. Once the stress of the accident is over and the person has calmed down, the blood pressure should go back to its normal level and be maintained at that level until the next period of stress. The diagnosis of high blood pressure is generally made when a person's blood pressure averages (stays) above the maximum of 140 over 90 on 3 blood pressure recordings taken at different times.

If you are uncertain about what your blood pressure should be, ask your physician. He or she will take into account your age, weight, body build, and level of activity to determine the boundaries your blood pressure should stay within.

Which of the 2 numbers of my blood pressure is most important?

Both the systolic and diastolic components of your blood pressure are important, but your physician will be most concerned with the lower number, or diastolic blood pressure. The resting diastolic pressure should stay below 90. If an average of several blood pressure records shows that your diastolic pressure stays at or above 90, then the diagnosis of high blood pressure can be made.

The systolic blood pressure is also important, but it normally elevates slightly with age as the arteries of the circulatory system get somewhat harder. A slightly higher systolic reading does not necessarily mean that an individual has significant high blood pressure; it is simply the normal course of things as a person ages.

SYMPTOMS

If I have high blood pressure, what symptoms might I experience?

Since your blood vessel system goes to every part of your body, high blood pressure will obviously affect your whole body. It's similar to your car's radiator when the pressure within it builds; the cap will hold for a while but eventually the cap is going to blow. When your blood pressure stays constantly elevated, you risk your body's blowing its top with a stroke, heart attack, or kidney disease.

But strangely enough, even with all that pressure, many people have absolutely no symptoms. In fact, the vast majority of people are stunned and confused when told that they have high blood pressure because they feel great. But there are some symptoms that are typically related to high blood pressure such as headaches, dizziness, or just generally not feeling well. The classic hypertension headache will be there when the person wakes up in the morning and often will gradually go away during the day. This is different from a tension headache that gets worse as the day progresses. People with hypertension might also experience ringing in the ears (tinnitus) or blurred vision. Again, I must emphasize that the vast majority of people with hypertension have no symptoms; they feel great. Whether you have symptoms or not, the seriousness of hypertension is still there. It must be treated.

HYPERTENSION

What is the difference between high blood pressure and hypertension?

Hypertension is a disease defined as "the persisent elevation of blood pressure." In most cases, the words *high blood pressure* and *hypertension* are synonymous.

According to the American Heart Association, hypertension affects an estimated 23 million Americans or 20% of the adult population. Of this 23 million, only 11 million are aware that they have hypertension. In other words, at least 50% of the people who have hypertension don't even know it. No wonder hypertension is called the silent killer.

Hypertension is a deadly problem. Uncontrolled hypertension can and does contribute to over 60,000 deaths annually by causing strokes, heart attacks, and heart failure. Hypertension is probably 1 of the most common chronic diseases in our country; it's also the easiest to detect. Having your blood pressure checked regularly can save your life.

Are some people more likely to have hypertension than others?

Hypertension can begin at any time, but it generally begins around age 30 and becomes increasingly common as people get older. Certain individuals are more likely to develop hypertension, and the following list describes some of them:

- If your mother or father had hypertension, you are more likely to develop hypertension in the future.
- Men are more frequently and severely affected than women.
- Blacks, especially black males, are more likely to have hypertension than the rest of the population.
- People who are overweight, especially of short stature, are more likely to develop hypertension.
- Pregnant woman or those who take birth control pills are more likely to develop hypertension.
- People who smoke, are under a great deal of stress, or do not get appropriate exercise are more likely to develop hypertension.

CAUSES

What causes high blood pressure?

For 90% of the people who have hypertension, there is no known cause. This type of hypertension is called essential hypertension. Some factors do seem to play a part in the development of essential hypertension: excessive weight, heavy salt intake, stressful lifestyle, and a family history of hypertension.

161

Only 5% to 10% of people who have hypertension have an underlying medical condition. If the underlying medical problem can be detected and corrected, then hypertension can be cured for this 5% to 10%.

Some of the medical conditions that can cause hypertension are diseases of the kidney, especially diseases related to the narrowing of the arteries leading from the body into the kidney (renal artery stenosis). Tumors of the adrenal glands can also cause high blood pressure by increasing the level of adrenalin and other chemicals throughout the body.

Another correctable cause of hypertension is a localized narrowing or coarctation of the aorta. In this congenital defect, a segment of the aorta, the body's largest artery, is narrowed so that the heart must work much harder to push blood through the narrowing. When this condition is corrected by surgery, the blood pressure will generally return to normal.

Certain unusual diseases of the nervous system such as brain tumors or infections of the brain (encephalitis) are also related to the development of high blood pressure. When the conditions are treated, the high blood pressure is brought under control.

Remember, though, that 90% of the people have no known cause of their hypertension and, therefore, no *cure*. Medications and medical treatment programs can keep the blood pressure under control, but these people will always have hypertension.

HEREDITY

Can hypertension be inherited?

Heredity seems to play an important role in the development of essential hypertension because this disorder occurs more often in people with a family history of high blood pressure. If 1 of your parents has the disease there is a 50% chance that you or a brother or sister will develop it, usually between the ages of 40 and 50, according to the American Heart Association. If both parents suffer from hypertension, the chance that 1 child will develop it rises to approximately 95%.

Of course, just because your parents have hypertension doesn't mean you will develop it. It does become more critical for you to make sure that all of the other potential causes of hypertension are reduced. If both parents have hypertension, you should make an extra effort to reduce your salt intake, exercise regularly, maintain an ideal body weight, stop smoking, and handle the stressful parts of your life as best you can. You can't do anything about heredity, but you can do something about the other contributing causes of hypertension.

TREATMENT

What are the 1st steps in treating high blood pressure?

When high blood pressure is diagnosed, your physician will recommend a program consisting of weight reduction, exercise, stress reduction, and salt restriction. If any other specific problems such as high cholesterol are present, other modifications in your diet will be recommended. If you smoke, your physician will strongly recommend that you stop. All of these modifications of lifestyle are used to try to lower your blood pressure without using medications. Depending upon the severity of your blood pressure, your physician may allow up to 2 to 3 months to see if these lifestyle changes actually cause any significant reduction in your blood pressure.

If my blood pressure is still elevated, will my physician recommend high blood pressure medicine?

If your blood pressure continues to be elevated despite lowering stress, losing weight, exercising, not smoking, and restricting salt, your physician will probably recommend starting you on medication for the control of the blood pressure. Hypertension medications combined with alterations in lifestyle can significantly reduce blood pressure. Probably 75% of persons with high blood pressure will require some form of medication. Most physicians will use a step-by-step approach, which means they will start with very small dosages of a single medication, increase the dose of that drug, and then add other medications until the blood pressure reaches the desired levels.

There are basically 4 steps your physician will need to consider in starting you on high blood pressure medication. During the 1st step, the physician may begin therapy by prescribing diuretics to help rid the body of excess salt and water. People who begin diuretics need to understand that they may urinate more frequently than usual. Examples of these medications are the thiazides and the potassium-sparing diuretics. Side effects are not terribly frequent, but if you experience weakness, fatigue, or stomach upset, tell your physician. He or she may need to adjust the dosage or change to a different medication.

If a physician finds that the diuretic alone does not control the patient's blood pressure, then as a 2nd step, he or she will probably suggest combining the diuretic with drugs such as reserpine, methyldopa, or a beta-blocking agent. These 3 medications work in different ways but, combined with diuretic therapy, can significantly lower blood pressure. (I must add here that beta-blocking agents are considered by some physicians as a step 1 medication. A beta-blocker can often be used by itself in the initial stage of treating hypertension.)

The 3rd step adds drugs that help dilate the blood vessels and increase the blood flow to the kidneys. Medications such as hydralazine can, therefore, be added to a diuretic or a step 2 drug for the additional control of blood pressure.

If medications in step 1 through 3 have not significantly reduced the blood pressure the physician may go to step 4 medications. These are the strongest drugs and will have the highest incidence of side effects. Guanethidine is an example of a step 4 medication.

Perhaps 50% of all newly diagnosed hypertensives can be controlled with step 1 medication. Another 25% can be controlled by adding step 2 medication. Only 15% to 20% will require step 3 drugs, and an even smaller percentage will need the addition of step 4 medications.

If I begin to take medication, will I ever be able to stop it?

Remember that hypertension is never cured, it is only treated. Of course, if other significant factors in your lifestyle change, the physician may be able to reduce or even eliminate some of the medications needed. But if your physician starts you on drugs for your high blood pressure, chances are that you will always be on them. Warning: Remember that if your physician starts you on medication for your high blood pressure, it is only treating the disease, not curing it. *Never* stop or alter the dosage of your hypertension medication without consulting your physician. If you are adequately controlled on high blood pressure medication and feel good, that doesn't mean that you can stop or reduce it by yourself. Stopping or reducing your medication without your doctor's okay is a dangerous, perhaps even deadly, practice.

TESTS

What laboratory tests will my physician use to determine the cause of my high blood pressure?

After a complete physical has been done and a history has been taken by your physician, he or she will probably want to order a series of simple laboratory tests. These tests help in eliminating some of the potentially curable causes of hypertension that we have discussed. The necessity of these tests is somewhat controversial since only 5% to 10% of people will have any of these problems, but almost all physicians agree that it is important to determine if you are in that 5% to 10%.

The 1st test would be a simple urinalysis to determine if any protein, blood, or sugar is in your urine. This could indicate the presence of diabetes or kidney disease. Your physician will also want to test your blood for the level of chemicals known as the blood urea nitrogen, or BUN. If this level is high, the test may indicate the presence of some underlying kidney disease, which could be the cause of your elevated blood pressure.

Another test your physician might perform checks the level of potassium in the blood. An abnormal potassium level could signal the presence of an adrenal tumor and could also indicate what treatment might be most effective for you.

Cholesterol has been shown to increase the risk of heart disease and is associated with people who have high blood pressure. Your physician will probably want to do a screening test to determine your level of cholesterol and perhaps other fats in your blood, such as triglycerides.

Depending upon your age and the findings of the blood and urine tests, your physician may want to order more detailed tests to evaluate your high blood pressure. An electrocardiogram and a chest x-ray may be important if there is any indication of underlying heart disease or weakening of the heart muscle.

The ability to effectively treat hypertension is directly related to the effects that hypertension has had on the organ systems of your body. The way in which hypertension affects your body will play a significant role in the type of treatment your doctor recommends.

IMPORTANCE OF POTASSIUM

Why do some people have to take potassium with their blood pressure medication?

As we have discussed, many people take diuretics for control of their blood pressure, and almost all diuretic medications have the additional side effect of eliminating potassium from the body.

Potassium is a critical element needed by all our cells, especially those in the heart, for proper functioning. The body can do without excess water and salt, but it can't do without potassium. Probably 50% to 75% of all people on diuretic medication will also have to take potassium supplements.

These supplements can be given through liquids, tablets, or effervescent powders. Regardless of which preparation your physician prescribes, make sure that you continue to take your potassium supplement as long as your physician directs.

People who take potassium supplements will also notice that their physician will want to check the potassium level in their blood periodically. This is to make sure that adequate amounts of supplements

165

are being taken to maintain a normal level of potassium in the blood system.

What are some of the possible symptoms of low potassium?

People who develop low blood potassium will experience generalized weakness, fatigue, and muscle cramping. They might also experience dizziness, especially when they get up or stand up quickly. If you are on high blood pressure medication and begin to develop any of these symptoms, consult your physician immediately.

Never begin taking potassium except under the strict supervision of your physician. Taking potassium without knowing exactly how much you should take is dangerous. Taking potassium that you buy over the counter or from a natural food store could lead to too much potassium in your blood—this is as serious a problem as not having enough.

"MILD" HIGH BLOOD PRESSURE

If I have only mild high blood pressure, do I really need treatment?

Diastolic blood pressure in the range of 90 to 104 has often been referred to as mild. Many people with mild hypertension felt that they really did not need any treatment. In fact, many physicians did not introduce treatment for people whose diastolic blood pressure ranged from 90 to 95.

Recent studies have shown, however, that the risk of many heart problems and of early death for people with so-called mild high blood pressure is more than 2 times that of people whose diastolic blood pressure stays below 90.

On the positive side, recent studies have also shown that the treatment of mild high blood pressure makes a significant difference in reducing early death and illness. There really is no such thing as mild high blood pressure anymore. Almost all blood pressure with a diastolic reading above 90 should be treated in some way by a physician.

PHYSICIAN-PATIENT COOPERATION

How can I help my doctor help me with my high blood pressure?

The treatment of hypertension must be a joint effort between physician and patient. The physician adds his or her medical expertise regarding the diagnosis and the selection of therapy for the control of blood pressure. But the patient has an equally important responsibility.

It is the patient's responsibility to follow explicitly the direction of the physician about making lifestyle changes and taking medication. The patient must also realize the importance of frequent follow-up visits to assure that the blood pressure gets under control and stays there. The patient should take medication exactly as the physician has prescribed: at no time stop medication, voluntarily change the dose, or take a neighbor's medication because it's supposed to "work better." Any change of medication or alteration of the therapy plan must be made in a joint decision by patient and physician.

If physician and patient live up to their responsibilities in the treatment of hypertension, there is no reason that each patient should not lead a long, productive life with a significant reduction in the chance of developing a stroke, a heart attack, or kidney disease.

11.

The Digestive System

FUNCTION

What function does the digestive system perform?

Your digestive system has a major function to perform in the body—to break down food that you eat into the vital nutrients essential for proper functioning. Food is broken down mechanically by chewing and chemically by the digestive juices into its simplest forms. Then these broken-down products are absorbed through the intestines into the blood. The blood system carries the nutrients to the rest of your body to provide energy and to rebuild and repair cells. The entire process, from chewing to absorption, is digestion.

The digestive tract is a 25′ tube, consisting of the mouth, esophagus, stomach, and small and large intestines. Once food has been chewed, it moves into the esophagus, the tube from the mouth into the stomach. The muscles of the esophagus continuously squeeze food down into the stomach. A valvelike muscle at the junction of the esophagus and the stomach keeps food and acid in the stomach. This junction, the lower esophageal sphincter, is extremely important in proper digestion.

When the chewed food reaches the stomach, it begins its breakdown into the vital nutrients, with the help of hydrochloric acid produced in the stomach. Your stomach can expand rather effortlessly to accept the food you've eaten and then slowly discharge it into the 1st portion of the small intestine—the duodenum. Further breakdown of the liquid food occurs within the duodenum when the food is mixed with special chemicals—bile from the liver and enzymes from the pancreas. The gallbladder forces bile into the duodenum to help with fat digestion. The pancreatic enzymes reduce the food into simpler components.

The small intestine seems inappropriately named, because it measures about 22'. But within that 22' of small intestine, the digestive enzymes and bile further break down food into the smaller components, so that by the time the food reaches the large intestine all of the components essential for our well-being have been absorbed through the lining of the small intestine into the blood.

The large intestine, also called the colon, is only approximately 3' long, but it is much wider than the small intestine. In the large intestine, most of the remaining water is removed from the undigested food, leaving only undigested material and enormous numbers of bacteria. This waste material, the stool or feces, is stored at the end of the large intestine, or rectum.

The same rhythmic muscle actions, peristalsis, that have pushed the food through the entire digestive system push the undigested food slowly into the rectum until enough accumulates to cause the sensation of needing to have a bowel movement.

STOMACHACHE

What causes stomachaches?

When someone complains of a stomachache, it means that there is pain somewhere in the area of the stomach or abdomen. However, many different things can cause stomachaches. Assuming a stomachache comes only from the stomach is incorrect and could lead to choosing the wrong medication to treat the pain. In general, stomachaches can result from a malfunctioning of many of the organs of the digestive system.

For most people, a stomachache means heartburn or indigestion. A much more serious problem that can cause a stomachache is an ulcer, which develops when the hydrochloric acid that breaks down food also "digests" a portion of the stomach lining.

Some people use the word *stomachache* to describe a cramping pain that comes in waves, reaching a peak and then subsiding. These pains usually originate further down in the digestive system, in the peristaltic action of the small or large intestine.

Most stomachaches disappear in a short period of time, but if the pain is severe, recurs, lasts more than 6 hours, or is associated with protracted nausea and vomiting, you should consult your physician.

INDIGESTION, HEARTBURN, AND BLOATING

Why do I have a lot of indigestion?

169

Indigestion means different things to different people, but it is usually a mild to fairly severe discomfort associated with a feeling of fullness or bloating, especially after eating. Indigestion can be caused by eating too much or too fast or by the stomach's failure to empty properly. Foods that irritate your stomach can also produce indigestion.

Obviously, the best solutions for intermittent indigestion are to eat slowly, eat well-balanced meals at regular times, and avoid overeating. Also try to identify specific foods that seem to bring on this feeling of fullness and bloating and eliminate them from your diet. If you've tried all of these solutions and the indigestion continues, consult your physician to see if there are any underlying causes that could be corrected.

What is heartburn?

Heartburn has nothing whatsoever to do with your heart. It occurs when the valve separating the esophagus and the stomach is not functioning properly. Normally, when food passes from the esophagus into the stomach, this valve will close, keeping the digested food and acid in the stomach. Occasionally, this undigested food and acid can pass back through the valve into the esophagus. Because the lining of the esophagus is very sensitive, the acid creates a burning sensation that you feel as being located right beneath your heart.

Heartburn can be treated in several ways. Avoid foods that bring on the heartburn. Very rich and spicy foods are often at fault as are alcoholic and caffeine-rich beverages. Smoking can also aggravate this condition because it increases the acid produced in the stomach.

Another way to relieve heartburn is to neutralize the acid in your stomach and soothe the lining of the esophagus by taking antacids after meals and at bedtime. However, if the heartburn continues, is associated with nausea or vomiting, or occurs upon exertion, you should see your physician immediately.

Are there ways to alleviate heartburn?

Some very simple measures may be surprisingly helpful in easing occasional heartburn. In general, these measures are designed to help the esophagus do its job more easily and to protect the muscles of the lower esophagus from substances that may weaken it. Certain foods such as fats, peppermint, and chocolate can weaken the muscles in the lower esophagus. Coffee and tomato or orange juice are very acidic and can also irritate the esophagus. Therefore, it is a good idea to avoid these substances or limit the amounts you take in.

Since heartburn is typically worse after meals, eating smaller meals and avoiding snacks will help a lot.

You may have noticed that lying down aggravates heartburn. This is because lying down negates the effect of gravity and lets the acid and food seep up into the esophagus. Don't lie down for about 1 to 2 hours after eating.

Excessive heartburn can be aggravated by being overweight or by wearing tight-fitting clothes. Losing weight and avoiding clothes that bind or pinch at the waist will help, also.

Why do I get a bloated feeling after meals?

The normal digestive process produces a good bit of gas as a by-product. Bloating occurs when too much of this gas accumulates in the stomach or the colon.

People who complain of excessive amounts of bloating may have a problem with the production of bile where the stomach and gallbladder don't quite coordinate. When this occurs, the normal passage of food through the intestines is disrupted and causes a buildup of food and gas.

Bloating is rarely serious, but it can produce severe pain. If you have a tendency to feel bloated after meals, you should avoid foods such as cauliflower, cabbage, and beans that produce a lot of gas. A high-fiber diet may also help to reduce bloating. If these simple measures do not work, ask your physician about medications that can be prescribed for this problem.

NAUSEA, VOMITING, AND DIARRHEA

What can I do at home if I develop nausea and vomiting?

Vomiting occurs when the valve between the stomach and the esophagus relaxes and the muscles of the abdomen tighten up. The pressure created by the tightening of the muscles forces the food from the stomach back up the esophagus and into the mouth.

A major cause of vomiting is gastroenteritis, a short-lived infection of the digestive system caused by a virus. This generally lasts 2 to 3 days and may be accompanied by fever and diarrhea. If you experience a sudden onset of nausea, vomiting, diarrhea, and a low-grade fever, you probably have viral gastroenteritis. Other causes of vomiting include food poisoning and severe anxiety.

The best way to treat the vomiting is to take away anything that stimulates or irritates the digestive system. Stop eating all solid foods and go on clear liquids, such as ginger ale, tea, or Gatorade.

Going on clear liquids should reduce the nausea and vomiting. With gastroenteritis, you may continue to have loose, runny stools, but as long as they are not producing severe cramping and subside within a day or so, there should be no problem.

Some over-the-counter medications can ease the symptoms of nausea and vomiting. Many medications for diarrhea also contain drugs to soothe your stomach and reduce nausea and vomiting. The most common are Pepto-Bismol, Donnagel, and Kaopectate.

Nausea and vomiting associated with diarrhea that lasts more than 4 or 5 days or is unresponsive to the above treatments should be reported to your physician.

What are some of the best ways to treat diarrhea in children?

Diarrhea or loose, runny stool is a problem that occurs frequently in young children. Diarrhea can be a symptom of anything from infections of the intestinal tract to ear and throat infections, teething, or even the common cold. This type of diarrhea often lasts only 2 or 3 days and can usually be treated without medication. But since small children are so susceptible to dehydration, at the 1st signs of progressive diarrhea, especially associated with vomiting, you need to start the following measures:

1. For 24 to 36 hours, give only clear liquids, such as soft drinks, tea, Gatorade, Pedialyte (available at the drugstore), or sugar water. Sugar water can be made by mixing 1 quart boiled water with 2 tablespoons sugar *and* a ½ teaspoon salt.

2. During the 2nd 24 hours, if the diarrhea is improving, you can begin plain gelatin, clear soups or broth, rice or barley cereal mixed with water, diluted fruit juices, ripe bananas, and dry toast or saltine crackers. If the diarrhea recurs, return to step 1 for the next 24 hours. (*Note:* Any time a child has vomiting or diarrhea, you should avoid milk and milk products. Also, do not give medications such as paregoric, Kaopectate, or antibiotics unless prescribed by your physician.)

3. On the 3rd day, if the diarrhea continues to improve, you may gradually add soft foods such as oatmeal, grits, or mashed potatoes.

4. On the 4th day, if the diarrhea has completely cleared up, the child can resume a normal diet, continuing to avoid excessive amounts of milk or milk products until the 5th or 6th day.

If your child is unable to take liquids because of vomiting, get in touch with your physician immediately.

CONSTIPATION

What causes occasional constipation?

172

As you know, waste materials pass into the colon (large intestine) and are pushed on toward the rectum by muscle contractions. By the time the waste material reaches the rectum, most of the water has been drawn out, and the waste material is fairly solid.

The contractions of the intestines cannot be controlled in the same way you control the movement of your arm. They are involuntary contractions but can be greatly affected by factors such as stress, illness, lower bowel habits, lack of exercise, inadequate amount of fluids, and diet.

When the peristaltic contractions in your bowel are sluggish, the waste material moves very slowly and the water is drawn out high up in the colon, causing the mass to become very hard and dry. This creates the problem of constipation.

How do you define constipation?

Constipation is a "condition characterized by infrequent bowel movements that are hard, dry, and difficult to pass." The key word is *infrequent,* a definition that will vary with each person. For some people, normal bowel habits mean 1 or more stools a day, while for others, a bowel movement every 2 to 3 days is normal. Experiencing a daily movement is *not* mandatory.

However, if *your* normal pattern becomes infrequent, and the stools are harder or drier than usual, then you are probably suffering from some degree of constipation.

How can I treat my constipation?

There are many causes of constipation. Some, like stress, are difficult to control, as are some illnesses. Usually the constipation connected with a specific stress or illness will subside when the stress or illness is gone.

The average person who develops constipation can best treat the problem through manipulation of diet. Foods that contain high levels of fiber provide the bulk that is essential for normal functioning of the colon. Without the necessary bulk in your diet, the colon may "sense" that there is no waste material to push through, and the normal intestinal contractions will slow down. Increasing the fiber in your diet can be accomplished by eating more bran, bran cereals, and fiber bread or by taking natural fiber materials found in some over-the-counter medications.

The use of laxatives for frequent constipation is not recommended and *can* be harmful. Although laxatives are often recommended by families when anyone develops constipation, self-medication with laxatives can create more problems than it solves. Most laxatives are harsh and force bowel movements. Laxatives can also be habit-forming and, if taken often, discourage the natural bowel contractions, making it necessary to take a laxative to have any bowel movement.

LAXATIVES

If my physician recommends a laxative, what kind should I choose?

Many types of laxatives can be purchased in the drugstore. The stronger laxatives produce a fairly unformed or fluid stool and include everything from castor oil, an old remedy, to some newer products. Saline laxatives (milk of magnesia or epsom salts) and contact laxatives (including phenolphthalein and bisacodyl) fall into this category. In hospitals, high dosages of strong laxatives are recommended only when people are about to undergo x-rays of the digestive system or similar tests.

Contact laxatives act on the lining of the lower colon and usually produce a soft or semisoft stool in approximately 2 to 8 hours. Some of these laxatives are chemicals, while others are extracts of herbs.

Another group of laxatives, including mineral oil, stool softeners, and bulk-forming agents, is considered to be more gentle. Most bulk-forming laxatives contain dietary fiber and produce a very gentle correction of the constipation. These are considered to be the 1st choice of treatment for people suffering from constipation. The most common bulk-forming laxative is psyllium hydrophilic mucilloid, sold as Metamucil or a similar product. This natural dietary fiber is refined from the psyllium seed and acts by holding large amounts of water and forming a gel that softens the stool, producing a bowel movement in 1 to 3 days.

HIGH-FIBER DIET

What are the benefits of a high-fiber diet?

Medical research shows that people who maintain high-fiber diets have a much lower incidence of colon problems. People who eat a great deal of fiber rarely have irritable bowel syndromes, diverticulosis, chronic constipation, hemorrhoids, or cancer of the colon. In fact, the American Cancer Society recommends a diet high in fiber to help in the prevention of colon cancer.

What kinds of foods can I eat to supplement my diet with fiber?

174

Eat more plant foods such as grains, beans, fruits, vegetables, nuts, and seeds. You will find a good deal of fiber in asparagus, kidney beans, navy beans, broccoli, brussels sprouts, cabbage, and raw or cooked eggplant.

Apples contain more fiber than almost all of the other fruits except blackberries and raspberries. Grapefruit, oranges, and pineapples have less fiber content.

Grain cereals, especially All-Bran, corn flakes, Wheaties, and Shredded Wheat, have lots of fiber in them. A bowl of any of these each morning will provide an adequate daily supply of fiber. Bran cereals have 5 to 6 times more fiber than whole wheat bread.

It's very important to eat the proper amount of fiber each day. If you haven't been aware of fiber, your diet changes may take some getting used to. Finding innovative ways to prepare high-fiber foods will increase your chances of sticking to the diet and decrease your chances of having future problems with your colon.

HEMORRHOIDS

What are hemorrhoids?

Reference has been made to hemorrhoids as far back as 2250 B.C., and through the ages hemorrhoids, often called piles, have plagued millions of people, including the Emperor Napoleon.

Hemorrhoids are simply enlarged, bulging (varicose) veins located in and around the rectum. The problems begin when these varicose veins become irritated, causing swelling, pain, itching, and bleeding.

Are all hemorrhoids the same?

The pain and the discomfort of hemorrhoids may be the same, but the types of hemorrhoids are not. The external hemorrhoid develops from the bulging and swelling of veins on the outside of the rectum. The bulging and swelling of internal hemorrhoids are hidden from view inside the lower portion of the rectum. When these hemorrhoids enlarge and protrude outward, they are called prolapsed hemorrhoids.

The pain associated with hemorrhoids is created when blood that gets congested in the enlarged vein begins to harden or clot, causing swelling.

Hemorrhoids can also cause frequent bleeding from the rectum. This occurs when hard stools pass over a hemorrhoid and cause a small cut or crack in its surface.

What is the best way to prevent hemorrhoids?

175

Most hemorrhoids are the result of an abnormality in the bowels—both constipation and diarrhea put an excessive amount of stress on the muscles and blood vessels around the rectum. These conditions also make the hemorrhoids uncomfortable once they have developed.

Be sensitive to your bowel functions, and answer the urge for a bowel movement promptly. If you delay having a bowel movement, you may have to strain later on to produce the bowel movement. Straining greatly increases the pressure in the lower rectum and can cause congestion of the veins, leading to hemorrhoids.

Also, following a diet high in fiber and increasing the amount of fluids you drink significantly reduce your chances of constipation and hemorrhoids.

If I have hemorrhoids, how can I treat them?

If you have developed hemorrhoids that are very small and not painful, the best way to treat them is keep them from getting any worse. Adjust your eating habits to increase the amount of fiber you have in your diet. You may also want to talk with your physician about a very mild stool softener that will decrease the pressure in the lower rectum.

If you have an acute attack of hemorrhoids with swelling and clotting in the veins, the 1st treatment is to sit in a hot sitz bath. The heat from the sitz bath contracts the hemorrhoids and reduces the swelling and the pain. Your physician can also recommend certain medications (such as hydrocortisone) to apply to the inside or outside of the rectum. These medications can significantly reduce the swelling and pain.

If your hemorrhoids bleed, you should consult your physician.

If your hemorrhoids do not respond to topical medication and heat, your physician may need to lance them. After the application of an anesthetic (Novocain), a small incision (cut) will be made in the hemorrhoids to release the clot. Once the clot is removed, the hemorrhoids are more likely to respond to heat and medication.

Hemorrhoids that continually reappear and are unresponsive to normal therapy may need to be surgically removed. This procedure, a hemorrhoidectomy, removes the affected veins. There is some degree of discomfort for a few days after this surgery, but it can lead to long-lasting relief.

12.

Special Diseases and Disorders of the Digestive System

ULCER

What is an ulcer?

Ulcers are small open breaks or craters in the lining of the upper digestive tract. Ulcers occur most often in the duodenum, the upper portion of the small intestine, and less commonly in the stomach itself.

Ulcers are created when the hydrochloric acid in the stomach eats away at the stomach or duodenum wall. If you picture dropping some acid on the back of your hand, you can visualize how it would begin to eat away at your skin and eventually create a cavity known as an ulcer. The same condition occurs in your stomach when, for a variety of reasons, the hydrochloric acid begins to eat away at the lining.

In general, ulcers are caused by an imbalance in the stomach because of too much stomach acid or a weakness in the stomach lining. This imbalance allows the stomach acids and enzymes to eat through the stomach's protective lining and produce the ulcers. However, there is not, as has been commonly thought, a direct relationship between excessive acid and ulcers. Many people who have ulcers secrete large amounts of acid, but other people with serious ulcers have normal amounts of acids.

Many experts, therefore, believe that another cause of ulcer formation is poor resistance within the tissue lining to the normal acid content of the stomach. Cigarette smoking, for instance, will interfere with the production of normal substances in the lining that help neutralize

177

some of the acid. Therefore, the ulcer produced from cigarette smoking is caused not by an excessive amount of acid but by a decrease in the ability of the lining to neutralize the acid.

How can I tell if I have an ulcer?

The primary symptom of an ulcer is pain generally centered in the pit of the stomach just below the rib cage. This pain follows a fairly characteristic pattern beginning several hours after eating or during the night when the stomach is empty. The pain can be described as a gnawing or aching sensation, but it may grow into a sharp stabbing or burning pain. Occasionally, there is no pain associated with an ulcer, and the symptom may be chronic belching or heartburn. Another classic symptom of an ulcer is pain that will generally get better with antacids, milk, or food.

If you have any of these symptoms, it does not mean that you have an ulcer, but it does mean that conditions are going on in your stomach that could potentially produce an ulcer. If you have any of these symptoms, you should try to neutralize the stomach acid through the use of antacid medications and change your diet to avoid hot, spicy, or greasy foods. You should immediately stop all aspirin or aspirin compounds. If you smoke, stop smoking.

If the symptoms do not go away with these simple measures, you should consult your physician for the appropriate test to determine whether or not the lining of your duodenum or stomach has an ulcer.

How can my physician determine if I have an ulcer?

Many times your physician can have a strong suspicion that you have an ulcer simply by what you tell him or her about the pain. People who have characteristic pain that gets better when they drink milk, take antacids, or put food in the stomach are in a very suspicious category. However, sometimes your physician may not be able to definitely tell you whether or not you have an ulcer without doing some appropriate testing.

The most common way to prove or disprove an ulcer is to x-ray the upper stomach and duodenum. Referred to as an upper GI test, these x-rays are taken after you have swallowed a chalky material called barium. The barium will go down through your esophagus into your stomach and duodenum, and it will outline the lining of the digestive tract. If there is any disruption in this lining, such as could be created by ulcers, your physician will be able to see it. X-rays can detect up to 70% of all ulcers.

Over the past several years, a newer and more effective test to identify ulcers has been developed—endoscopy. In this procedure, a specialist in stomach disorders (a gastroenterologist) will pass a flexible tubing through your mouth down your esophagus into your stomach. This tube allows direct visualization of the lining of the stomach and duodenum. Through this flexible tube, the gastroenterologist can scan the whole lining of your stomach and duodenum and directly see any problems. Even though it sounds horrible, you will probably be given a sedative and have little discomfort.

If my physician finds that I have an ulcer, what treatment will be used?

The 1st stage of treating any ulcer condition is changing dietary habits. All foods that could potentially irritate an ulcer must be stopped. Years ago we used to put people on strict diets consisting of baby food and milk. We now know that we don't have to be quite as strict with the diet, but there are some obvious things that individuals with ulcers should avoid.

Anyone who has developed an ulcer should avoid hot, spicy, or greasy foods. All of these are known to increase the normal production of acid and thus complicate an ulcer condition. Patients should also stop drinking alcoholic beverages and certainly stop smoking. All medications that could potentially cause or irritate an already existing ulcer should also be stopped. This includes all medications containing aspirin or aspirin compounds and many of the newer medications used to treat arthritis. You would be amazed at how many over-the-counter medications contain aspirin.

After changing the diet and stopping any causative foods and medicines, your physician will probably place you on an antacid. Antacids come in either liquid or tablet form and are used to help neutralize the acid your stomach is currently producing. Most people will take the medication after meals and every couple of hours between meals.

Antacids differ in many ways. Some are fortified with simethicone and are beneficial in helping reduce the formation of gas. Some can cause diarrhea while others can cause constipation. If you have high blood pressure you have to watch the salt content of these medications. Your physician can tell you which antacid is best for your particular condition.

Next your physician will probably recommend a medication that can significantly reduce the amount of acid you produce. Several new medications on the market have an effect on decreasing your normal production of acid, especially when taken before meals and at bedtime.

Therefore, the treatment of an ulcer condition consists of diet, antacids, and medications. But there is an important part of the treatment that I have left out so far. Many people who suffer from ulcers are under a great deal of personal or emotional stress. Stress reduction is a very important part of the overall therapy. Recommendations such as counseling, exercise programs, and stress-reduction techniques have helped many to heal more quickly and to avoid recurrences.

Are there any new medications that can help ulcers?

There are 2 new medications on the market that have significantly increased our ability to help people with ulcers. The discovery of cimetidine and ranitidine, which cut down on the flow of digestive acids and enzymes permitting ulcers to heal, has markedly changed our success rate. Another new medicine for the treatment of ulcers is sucralfate, which forms a protective coating over the ulcer and gives it a chance to heal.

Many older drugs remain a valuable part of ulcer therapy, particularly the antacids. Antacids not only relieve the discomfort but actually promote the healing of duodenal ulcers. Selected individuals can also be treated with agents know as anticholinergics, drugs that slow down the stimulation of acid in the stomach. In any case, treatment of ulcers is tailored to the specific needs of each person.

What are some of the complications I can have from ulcers?

If you do not take care of your ulcer and if you fail to follow your physician's directions, bleeding is a serious complication. Bleeding can show itself as bright red vomit or black tarry stools. If you are bleeding from an ulcer, the blood in your stomach can combine with acid, forming a black coffeelike material. If this is thrown up, we refer to it as coffee-ground vomitus. If this material passes on through the digestive system, it can turn your stools black. The symptoms of bleeding are weakness and fatigue or, in cases of severe hemorrhage, loss of consciousness and shock.

Another serious complication occurs when the ulcer actually bursts, letting acid flow deep into the intestinal cavity. This acid can irritate the intestinal cavity and, along with bacteria, cause serious infection. If your ulcer bursts or perforates, your condition becomes a medical emergency requiring immediate surgery. A perforated ulcer causes the pain to be sudden and intense, and even the slightest movement seems to make it worse.

A bleeding ulcer does not mean that you will have to undergo surgery, but it is a serious complication. It means that you and your physician must work hard to dramatically reduce the acid production, stop the bleeding, and speed the healing process.

HIATAL HERNIA

What is a hiatal hernia?

In the normal digestive system is an area at the lower portion of the esophagus that functions as a valve to keep food in the stomach. A hiatal hernia occurs when that normal valve becomes loose and widens. Once it widens, it does not function properly, and acid and digested food can pass freely up through the valve into the lower esophagus. This is referred to as reflux and creates burning sensations in the upper stomach and under the breastbone. Generally, people will experience heartburn, gas, belching, and a feeling that food regurgitates into the back of the throat. Another common symptom is the feeling of hot acid or fluid in the back of the throat.

Hiatal hernias tend to occur in people who are over 50 years of age and in people who are overweight. Individuals with hiatal hernias often have heartburn after they eat, especially when they lie down after meals. When a person is standing, gravity will prevent some of this reflux, but upon lying down there is almost an open passage for food and acid to pass back up into the esophagus.

How can I tell whether or not my symptoms are from a hiatal hernia?

Probably the best way to tell whether or not you have a hiatal hernia is to be evaluated by your physician. Many times simply taking a complete history reveals the obvious diagnosis. However, if your physician is unsure or wants more definite tests, a barium study of the esophagus and stomach (upper GI series) can be performed. As barium flows down the esophagus and enters into this dilated valve, it can often be seen on x-rays.

What is the best way to treat a hiatal hernia?

Hernias can occur in other portions of the body and can be corrected by surgery. However, it is extremely rare to surgically treat a hiatal hernia. The best way to treat a hiatal hernia is to follow some simple steps to reduce the reflux of acid into the esophagus and neutralize the acid present.

181

Step 1. You should change your diet to avoid all types of food that will increase the acid production of the stomach. If you normally consume coffee or alcohol, chocolate or fatty foods, greasy foods or spicy foods, these should be stopped.

Step 2. You should avoid bending or stooping after eating since this can force food into the esophagus and cause heartburn.

Step 3. You should eat smaller but more frequent meals during the day, trying to avoid the foods listed above at all times.

Step 4. You should avoid lying down or reclining in a chair for up to 4 hours after eating.

Step 5. Refraining from smoking can significantly reduce the amount of acid produced.

Step 6. You should avoid tight clothing such as tight belts or girdles, which will increase the pressure in your stomach and thus increase your symptoms.

Step 7. If you are overweight, a great many of the symptoms of hiatal hernia can be reduced by reducing your weight.

Step 8. If you have major problems at night when you go to bed you should sleep with the head of your bed raised about 6″ to 8″ on firmly secured blocks.

Step 9. You should take antacids after each meal and at bedtime to reduce the acid in the stomach and thus the potential of reflux.

DIVERTICULOSIS AND DIVERTICULITIS

What is diverticulosis?

Diverticulosis is almost nonexistent in many parts of the world, such as India and Africa, but it is 1 of the most common bowel problems in the United States. Though diverticulosis is not a serious condition, more than 25% of Americans over the age of 40 have it as will about 50% of our population who reach 70 years of age.

Diverticulosis is derived from the Latin word *diverticulum*, which means "a small diversion from the normal path." Diverticulosis is created when balloonlike sacs or pouches (diverticula) develop in the walls of the large intestine. These tiny pouches are formed because of years of pressure exerted in the colon, creating weak spots. As the pressure builds over the years, these weak spots balloon out much as the tip of a balloon will. *Diverticulosis* is the term used to indicate that these pouches are present.

Often people with diverticulosis have no symptoms or, at the very most, a history of constipation and occasional cramping in the lower stomach. Bouts of constipation that alternate with diarrhea in a person over 50 could indicate diverticulosis.

What is diverticulitis?

When 1 of these pouches gets plugged up with waste material and becomes inflamed and infected, a condition known as *diverticulitis* is produced. Diverticulitis is characterized by episodes of fever and a crampy, colicky pain in the colon area. People with diverticulitis often have severe constipation; however, others will have rather frequent diarrhea.

Many times people with diverticulitis need to be hospitalized and placed on intravenous fluids so the colon can rest. They will also be placed on specific antibiotics to reduce the infection. A serious complication of diverticulitis occurs when an area begins to bleed. Bleeding from diverticulitis can create bright red blood from the rectum or, more rarely, black stools. The bleeding must be identified and controlled, or anemia can develop.

Perhaps the most serious complication occurs when 1 of these balloons or pouches bursts. Then the contents of the colon empty into the open abdominal cavity, creating a serious infection called peritonitis.

Is there any way that I can avoid excess pressure in my colon and thus reduce my chances of developing diverticulosis?

Constipation is the primary cause for excess pressure in the colon. When the colon has to push hard, dry waste material, it must use extra force, thus creating extra pressure. This is much like the extra force needed to squeeze out toothpaste when the tube is almost empty.

If you can prevent constipation through the years, you can significantly reduce this chronic pressure and thus your chances of developing diverticulosis. A word of caution: The chronic use of laxatives can irritate the colon and weaken the walls. Therefore, constipation should be prevented through the use of bulk-forming laxatives such as those described earlier.

SPASTIC COLON

What is spastic colon?

Spastic colon is another name for perhaps the most common digestive tract disorder—irritable bowel syndrome. An estimated 22 million people suffer from irritable bowel syndrome, and ⅔ of them are women.

Irritable bowel syndrome is not a single disease but a group of symptoms. These symptoms include abdominal pain, which generally comes in waves, and altered bowel habits, such as diarrhea, constipation, or constipation alternating with diarrhea. Irritable bowel syndrome is most commonly associated with emotional stress and poor dietary habits.

The colon's ability to function normally is controlled by the body's nervous system. There are nerve impulses that stimulate the colon to contract and others that cause it to relax. When a fine balance between these 2 types of nerve impulses occurs, the gastrointestinal contents are pushed through the colon normally and painlessly.

In people with irritable bowel syndrome, this delicate balance of nerve impulses is disrupted. In addition to the regular contractions (peristalsis), irregular contractions occur that can upset the normal rhythm.

Constipation occurs when the peristaltic movements are inhibited, and diarrhea results when the nerve impulses to the colon are stimulated. The abdominal pain and cramping result from actual spasms within the colon and the gas buildup that can occur.

What things seem to trigger attacks of spastic colon?

Irritable bowel syndrome can be caused by a variety of conditions. Perhaps the most common are emotional upsets such as anxiety, stress, or depression. If a physician measures the strength of the contractions in the colon in people who are under stressful conditions, they will be much greater than in people who are relatively calm.

Dietary abuses also tend to make the spasms worse. Meals that are high in calories and fat content tend to produce exaggerated contractions in people with irritable bowel syndrome and lead to cramps and diarrhea. Fats in the form of oils and animal fats or even butter can stimulate severe attacks.

What treatment is available for people with irritable bowel syndrome?

Irritable bowel syndrome doesn't threaten your life, only your lifestyle. It is very important for people who have irritable bowel syndrome to be placed on a proper diet, generally high in fiber content. If enough fiber cannot be obtained in the diet, people will be placed on a supplement such as Metamucil. They also need to avoid the foods that are known to increase spasms.

Because of the tremendous amount of underlying emotional anxiety in most people with irritable bowel syndrome, proper therapy should include counseling and stress-reduction techniques. Medications prescribed by your physician can help lessen the nerve stimulation in the colon; 2 of the most common are tranquilizers and antispasmodics. Tranquilizers are used to help calm you down and thus take away many of the emotional triggers. Antispasmodics aid in returning normal colon contractions by stimulating chemicals that produce normal rhythm patterns.

INFLAMMATORY BOWEL DISEASE

What is the difference between spastic colon and colitis?

Spastic colon is a complex of symptoms related to simple spasms within the colon. Colitis, however, implies inflammation of the colon, and is in the category of disease referred to as inflammatory bowel disease.

Inflammatory bowel disease is not a single disease; it encompasses a variety of inflammations that can occur within both the small and the large colon. The inflammation of the lining of the wall is the common denominator that links all of these groups.

Proctitis tends to be very mild, is more common in middle-aged people, and often subsides spontaneously. In this disease, there is an inflammation in the lining of the colon from the rectum up into the lower portion of the large colon (the sigmoid colon).

Chronic ulcerative colitis occurs more often in younger people and frequently is seen for the 1st time in the late teens or early 20's. Chronic ulcerative colitis is a condition in which small ulcers are scattered throughout the colon.

Crohn's disease of the bowel differs significantly from the diseases described above. The inflammatory process involves not only the lining but also the wall of the bowel. This disease is characterized by intermittent bouts of nausea, vomiting, chills, fever, and abdominal pain.

What are some causes of inflammatory bowel disease?

Although research has been done for years to discover the exact causes of many of these inflammatory bowel diseases, no specific reasons have been found. There is no evidence that inflammatory bowel disease is inherited, although it does tend to occur more frequently in the Jewish population. Although emotional stress can occur in inflammatory bowel disease, there is no evidence that anxiety or emotional stress plays a primary role. We simply do not know why many people get inflammatory diseases of the bowel.

What are some of the symptoms of colitis?

A number of symptoms are fairly characteristic of the many forms of inflammatory bowel disease. The most common symptoms associated with them include the following:

- *Diarrhea*. Diarrhea or the frequent passage of stools is almost universally found in people with a form of inflammatory bowel disease. The stool may contain blood or an excessive amount of mucus. It is thought that the diarrhea results from an inflammation of the lining of the colon wall.
- *Pain*. Pain in the form of abdominal cramps most often occurs in the lower portion of the abdomen and is thought to be caused by both the inflammation and the spasm it creates. In Crohn's disease of the small bowel, for instance, crampy abdominal pain may be the 1st symptom and may be present before the diarrhea occurs.
- *Nausea and/or vomiting*. These symptoms are common in any digestive disease in which there is inflammation, and they are especially prominent in forms of colitis.
- *Weight loss*. Weight loss is a common symptom of inflammatory bowel disease, probably because people who suffer from intermittent bouts are taking in less calories. But it also may be due to the fact that the inflamed bowel simply does not function properly and cannot absorb the proper nutrients.
- *Anemia*. Low blood iron, or anemia, is thought to result from the inflammatory process that causes a constant oozing of blood from the inflamed bowel wall.
- *Fever*. Fever is quite common and in many instances differentiates inflammatory bowel disease from some of the less serious colon problems.

What is the treatment for colitis?

Colitis in all its forms tends to be a chronic disorder and, therefore, requires long-term therapy. It is very important for people with colitis to get adequate rest, nutritious diet, and regular exercise. In addition, they should try to avoid other infections, which can cause the colitis to worsen.

Since the cause of colitis is unknown, there is no specific treatment. Individuals with acute bowel disease who have diarrhea, fever, and bloody stools are generally treated in the hospital. The 1st approach is to put the colon at rest by not allowing the person to eat or drink and by administering intravenous fluids.

A number of medications that can be used in acute episodes can help a great deal. Steroids are frequently prescribed on a short-term basis to reduce severe inflammation. Other medications, such as Azulfidine, have also been found to be highly effective in reducing inflammation and keeping it from recurring. The advantage of Azulfidine is that it can be used over a long period of time. Recently, it has been found that Flagyl, a medication used in certain other types of infections, has had some benefit. Once the acute inflammation is brought under control, many people will have to be on 1 or both of these medications for a long period of time to reduce the possibility of recurrence.

If I have a form of colitis, is a normal lifestyle difficult?

Certainly not. If you have a form of colitis, proper diagnosis and treatment can allow you to lead a normal lifestyle. Since diarrhea is the most common symptom, proper diet and medication can enable you to travel at will.

However, people with colitis must pay particular attention to their overall health. Following a strict diet, exercising frequently under your physician's direction, and continuing to take your medications as long as they are prescribed are all excellent ways to live a normal lifestyle with colitis.

13.

Problems of the Genitourinary System

PROSTATE GLAND

Why do so many men have problems with the prostate gland?

All men have a prostate gland, and many will have problems with it at some time in their lives. The prostate gland is located just below the bladder at the very base of the penis, and it produces the milky fluid, or semen, that sperm live in.

The most common prostate problem, which can occur at any age, is an inflammation or infection of the gland, referred to as prostatitis. This infection can cause pain or discomfort at the base of the penis, increased frequency of urination, and some burning on urination. If a physician checks your prostate gland and finds it to be swollen and tender, he or she can usually cure the problem by using appropriate antibiotics.

Another problem with the prostate occurs in older men. Almost from the moment of birth, the prostate begins to enlarge. If a man lives long enough, his prostate can get large enough to close off or squeeze the urethra. This condition, benign prostatic hypertrophy, can cause a more frequent need to urinate, a change in the force and control of the urinary stream, and difficulty with erections. When these symptoms occur and become severe enough to interfere with normal urination, the enlarged prostate gland must be removed or scraped in a surgical procedure.

Can cancer occur in the prostate gland?

Prostate cancer is the 3rd leading type of cancer in men, just behind lung cancer and colon cancer. When present, the cancer starts near the outside of the prostate gland, and a physician can feel the cancerous nodule during a normal rectal examination. Although cancer of the prostate can cause an inability to urinate well, it usually does not.

Symptoms of prostate cancer can be minimal, and many men will not know that they have it unless they have a yearly prostate exam done by their physician.

KIDNEY STONE

What causes a kidney stone?

Kidney stones form when various chemicals congeal or crystallize within the urinary system. The majority of these will form within the kidney itself, then drop down into the ureter, the tube leading from the kidney to the bladder. As they travel down the small ureter, they will eventually reach a spot where they are larger than the tube and will become lodged. When this happens, they cause tremendous spasms of the ureter, severe intermittent pain, and difficulty with urination.

Kidney stones occur in about 5% of the population and are responsible for about 1 out of every 1000 hospitalizations. Men are 4 times more likely to have kidney stones than women, and whites are more frequently affected than blacks.

A person with a kidney stone will complain of a dull ache on 1 side that will begin to move around the front and down into the lower side of the abdomen. At some point, the pain will change from a dull ache to a severe intermittent pain, and it will radiate and feel as if it is moving down into the groin.

If I have had kidney stones, how can I prevent them from recurring?

Most people who have had kidney stones will average more than 3 attacks in their lifetime. Because of this, it is important to understand some of the ways to reduce the chances of having another attack. The stones are often made up of calcium, so it's important for "stone-formers" to reduce their intake of calcium by limiting their milk and milk product intake. They should also be checked for a high uric acid level in their blood, since this type of acid can form kidney stones (as well as gout). People with high uric acid levels will need medication to bring the acid level back to normal.

People who have had kidney stones can lead normal, healthy lives, but they must understand that a new stone can appear suddenly and without warning.

14.

Bone, Muscle, and Joint Problems

ARTHRITIS

What is arthritis?

Arthritis is probably 1 of the oldest known ailments. Writings from the ancient Greek and Roman civilizations record its presence. Ancient Egyptian mummies also show signs of arthritis. Today, things aren't much different. Over 50 million Americans suffer from some form of arthritis—about 25% of the population.

The word *arthritis* means "inflammation of the joint." Your joints are those structures formed when 2 or more bones come together. For instance, your knee is not a separate bone; it is a joint formed where the upper bone of the leg, the femur, comes together with the 2 lower bones of the leg, the tibia and the fibula.

Arthritis is different from the common complaint of arthralgia, or pain in the joints. With arthritis, there is pain plus some evidence of inflammation in the form of swelling, redness, warmth, or actual destruction in the lining of the joint. With arthralgia, the pain is present, but the inflammation is not. If the pain in your joints persists or is associated with any of the symptoms of inflammation, you may be suffering from 1 of over 100 different types of arthritis.

Is arthritis a disease of only older people?

The 2 most common types of arthritis are rheumatoid arthritis and osteoarthritis. It is true that osteoarthritis generally occurs in older people, but rheumatoid arthritis can affect persons of all ages.

A special condition known as juvenile rheumatoid arthritis severely affects the joints of very young children, and it is often crippling. So, arthritis is not a disease of the elderly; it can affect people of all ages.

If I have pain and stiffness in my joints, does that mean I have arthritis?

No matter what your age, if you wake up some morning with pain and stiffness in your joints, your 1st reaction may be that you are developing arthritis. However, this is usually not the case. Most of us will suffer occasional aching or stiffness in our joints from sleeping wrong or over-using our joints. This type of discomfort is occasional, generally short-lived, and responds to direct heat to the joint and rest for the joint. The vast majority of people who suffer from these aches and pains are not going to develop arthritis.

Another common complaint occurs when you wake up with some stiffness in your fingers. You may be convinced that this must be the same type of arthritis your grandmother had. Again, most of us will have this occasional stiffness; unless it persists over a long period of time and is associated with decreased ability to move the fingers or redness, swelling, and warmth in the joint, it is not an indication that you have or might develop arthritis.

However, 50 million Americans do have some form of arthritis. If any of these symptoms occur repeatedly and seem to persist for long periods of time, you should consult your physician to see if you have a form of arthritis. But for occasional stiffness in the joints, the best treatment is to apply heat (heating pad or warm to semihot water) and take an occasional dose of aspirin, if you are not sensitive to it.

I know I got my "bad heart" from my parents, but where did my arthritis come from?

We still do not know exactly why people develop arthritis. The 2 most common forms—osteoarthritis and rheumatoid arthritis—seem to have a tendency to run in families, but there is no direct evidence that the disease is inherited. However, gout is a form of arthritis that is passed on from generation to generation. (We'll discuss gout and its basis in heredity later in the chapter.)

The vast majority of people who suffer from some form of arthritis do not inherit the disease but develop it for reasons we haven't yet discovered. We do know that some predisposing conditions make people more prone to develop it. Obesity or being overweight is certainly a leading cause of persistent inflammation of the joints. It stands to reason that a person walking around with 50 to 75 extra pounds will have more stress placed on the joints, especially those of the lower leg. People who are sedentary and do not get exercise can develop pain and inflammation of the joints simply from inactivity. So, excluding gout, you can do something to lessen your chances of developing arthritis in the future: maintain your ideal body weight and exercise to keep the joints mobile.

Are all forms of arthritis basically the same?

No. All forms of arthritis have only 1 thing in common—inflammation of the joints. The ages at which you can be affected, the degree of destruction of the joint, the potential for being incapacitated, and the treatments are entirely different.

For instance, osteoarthritis primarily affects the elderly population and is associated with progressive difficulty in movement. Rheumatoid arthritis affects people of all ages, even young children, teenagers, and young adults. Gout primarily affects men and seems to be limited to specific joints of the body. It can be easily controlled with proper medication.

It is very important for you and your physician to find out what specific type of arthritis you have so that a treatment plan can be developed to fit your age and your particular condition.

OSTEOARTHRITIS

What is osteoarthritis?

Where 2 movable bones meet, they will form a union or a joint. The major joints in our bodies are those at the shoulders, elbows, wrists, fingers, hips, knees, ankles, and feet.

Where bones come together, they are covered by a smooth rubbery substance called cartilage. It acts as a cushion or shock absorber so that the bones don't rub together when the joint moves. The cartilage is kept well lubricated with a sticky substance called synovial fluid. By making the smooth cartilage slippery, this fluid helps the joint move smoothly.

Osteoarthritis occurs when the smooth cartilage begins to break down and become thinner. When this happens, the tips of the bones actually rub together, causing pain. The tips of the bones then break down, and little jagged bony lumps, called spurs, are formed.

The combination of worn cartilage, thicker bone surfaces, and the presence of spurs causes pain and inflammation around the joint—osteoarthritis.

Why does osteoarthritis occur mostly in older people?

We're not exactly sure, but it is generally believed that osteoarthritis is brought about by the wear and tear that occurs in the joints over the years. Each joint moves millions of times throughout someone's life. In some people, this constant movement causes a wearing down of the cartilage cushion in later life.

How can I tell if I am developing osteoarthritis?

The 1st symptoms of osteoarthritis are very subtle and may begin with only stiffness and swelling in the joints of the hands. The specific joints affected by the osteoarthritis most often are the joints where the fingers join the hand itself. Osteoarthritis can also cause stiffness in the last finger joint and, in early stages, may form nodules known as Heberden's nodes. These nodules, caused by the knobby bone spurs developing in that joint, can become tender and swollen.

Another common symptom of progressing osteoarthritis is muscle fatigue. Because of the changes within the joint, the muscles that support it have to work much harder and thus tire more easily.

As the disease progresses, deformities may develop in the joint because of the wearing down of the bone ends and the formation of bone spurs. Many times, people with osteoarthritis have swelling in the joints, especially the knees. This swelling, along with the pain, is the major reason why people with osteoarthritis are incapacitated.

If I have any of these symptoms, should I see my doctor?

Immediately. If you are having any of these symptoms and are over the age of 50, you should consult your physician for a proper diagnosis. Remember, there are over 100 different forms of arthritis. To properly treat the type you have, your physician must find out which one you have.

The best treatment for osteoarthritis is early detection. It can be detected through an examination of the joints themselves and through x-rays, but in the early stages of the disease, the primary diagnosis comes from the type of discomfort you have and its response to certain treatment.

If I have osteoarthritis, how should it be treated?

In the treatment of osteoarthritis, the 1st thing to remember, unfortunately, is that there is no cure. Many people believe that a drug, a pill, or an injection will cure their problem, but this is not the case. Nevertheless, the symptoms of osteoarthritis can be alleviated in many people, and the affected joint can be maintained at a relatively normal level of functioning.

The primary goals for the treatment of osteoarthritis are to relieve the pain and discomfort, to increase the use of the joint as much as possible, and to try to prevent further damage.

Anti-inflammation medicines, the most common of which is aspirin, can help relieve the pain of osteoarthritis. In individuals who can tolerate it, proper doses of aspirin help relieve the inflammation and return some degree of mobility to the joint. Other drugs, such as nonsteroidal anti-inflammatory medicines, which require prescriptions, essentially work like "high-powered" aspirin to relieve discomfort.

Exercise is also critical in the treatment of osteoarthritis. An exercise program tailored to your specific age and extent of disease can improve the motion of the joint and the strength of the muscles around it.

Heat is another important part of treatment. Taking hot baths or applying a heating pad can ease the pain of inflammation and relax tense, tired muscles. Finally, resting the entire body and the joints affected by osteoarthritis is extremely important. Trying to "keep going" may do more harm than good.

The treatment of osteoarthritis is a combined approach of all these therapies and is done with cooperation between the physician and the patient.

If I develop osteoarthritis, will it get worse? Will I be crippled?

It is really hard to say how the disease will progress. In many cases, it remains a very mild problem, causing only occasional pain and immobility. But in others, the disease progresses to the point that the joints actually degenerate and do not function properly. When you develop osteoarthritis, no one can predict the category you will fit in, and no one can say for sure whether your osteoarthritis will continue as it is, gradually get better, or grow worse.

We do know, however, that the best chance of lessening disability in the future comes from a well-designed treatment plan. It will take time, patience, and work, but the proper combination of medicine, heat, rest, and exercise will place you in the best position to prevent further disability.

Are there any side effects associated with the medicines used with osteoarthritis?

There are certain side effects with almost any medication, and those used to treat osteoarthritis are no exception. Remember that the drugs used are anti-inflammation medicines that specifically reduce the inflammation at the joint surface, reduce the swelling, and relieve the discomfort.

The prototype of this type of medication is aspirin. There are a few people who are simply allergic to aspirin, and they develop palpitations, wheezing, or fainting spells when they take it. Obviously, if these people have osteoarthritis, aspirin cannot be used. For another group of people, the major side effect is stomach upset. A burning sensation created in the stomach by the acid in the aspirin can be a potential problem; therefore, aspirin should always be taken with meals and at bedtime with a glass of milk. Never take aspirin on an empty stomach. In fact, most physicians usually recommend that patients take either a coated aspirin or 1 that is combined in tablet form with Maalox.

The other type of medication used in the treatment of osteoarthritis is the nonsteroidal anti-inflammatory drug. These drugs have side effects much like aspirin, so people taking these medications (Motrin, Feldene, Nalfon, Naprosyn, and others) should take them only on a full stomach and at bedtime with a glass of milk. The meals and milk help decrease the chance that the drugs will irritate the stomach. Other frequent side effects are abdominal cramping and diarrhea. If you experience any of these, consult your physician immediately so that the dosage or the medication can be changed.

I've heard that too much aspirin can cause bleeding ulcers.

Certainly, there are potential side effects from aspirin, especially since 6 to 8 a day must be taken to provide relief from the symptoms of arthritis. However, if aspirin is taken correctly and in the proper doses, chances are that you will have few, if any, side effects.

If you are taking more aspirin than your body can handle, you will probably have a slight ringing in your ears (tinnitus). If this happens, tell your physician about it immediately so that he or she can adjust the dosage. Your ears will ring *long* before you develop bleeding ulcers. But if you develop a burning sensation in your stomach, feel nauseous after taking aspirin, or have unusual abdominal cramping, consult your physician so that any potential problems from the aspirin can be found early and quickly resolved.

What types of exercise can I do if I have bad arthritis?

Exercise and rest are very important parts of the treatment of osteoarthritis. Used together and in the right combination, they will help keep your joints mobile and free of pain. Exercise serves 2 main purposes: it keeps the joints of your body moving and prevents them from freezing or staying in 1 position too long; and it strengthens the muscles that surround the joints, giving you better protection and support.

There are many different types of exercise that can help a person with osteoarthritis. The basic kind is the range-of-motion exercise. You move each joint in your body—back and forth, up and down, from side to side, and in almost every other position—taking each motion as far as it can go without creating pain.

A very good exercise for people with osteoarthritis is walking. If you do not have severe deformities of the hips or knees, walking for 15 to 20 minutes each day, swinging your arms and moving your neck while you walk, can give you a good workout. Other good exercises are swimming, supervised dancing, and supervised riding of a stationary bike.

Even if your joint deformities are so severe that your range of motion is tremendously limited, you can still do some exercises at home. Simply sitting in your chair each day and moving all the joints that you can possibly move for 15 to 20 minutes can help. It doesn't sound like much, but any exercise will help to keep some motion in your joints.

Remember that exercise, no matter how much or how little you are able to do, should be combined with the application of heat and frequent rest periods. Don't overdo! Your physician may also recommend that you see an exercise specialist known as a physical therapist. This person is trained to devise and help you execute a program that meets your special needs.

RHEUMATOID ARTHRITIS

What is rheumatoid arthritis?

Rheumatoid arthritis is an inflammation of the joint, just like osteoarthritis. But in rheumatoid arthritis, the inflammation begins in the synovial lining, the lining of the joint capsule. This lining begins to swell, the inflammation spreads to the cartilage and other parts of the joint, and the joint lining and cartilage are eventually destroyed. When this happens, the tips of the bones become covered by scar tissue instead of this protective lining, making the joint very rigid, swollen, and incapable of normal motion.

We don't know exactly why certain people develop rheumatoid arthritis or what causes it. It is not, as many people believe, caused by cold or damp climates, although the weather can influence its symptoms. It is not thought to be hereditary, even though it does appear to occur more often in certain families. Some experts believe that rheumatoid arthritis may be caused by a virus, and a great deal of research is being done in that area. While there are no definitive answers yet about the cause, we do know that rheumatoid arthritis often begins before the age of 40 and that women are affected 3 times more often than men. The diagnosis of rheumatoid arthritis is made by combining the characteristic symptoms and joint involvement with a blood test that can detect the disease.

What are some of the symptoms of rheumatoid arthritis?

In the very early stages, rheumatoid arthritis often causes only temporary pain, swelling, and tenderness in the joints, especially the hands, wrists, and feet. Osteoarthritis affects mostly the large joints; rheumatoid arthritis affects mainly the smaller joints.

Later on, these symptoms can actually go away, giving the individual a false sense of being "cured." Rheumatoid arthritis characteristically has periods of remission lasting for weeks, months, or even years, but it will usually reappear, often with more severe pain and inflammation than before.

As rheumatoid arthritis continues to progress, other symptoms of the disease may be found. In some people, rheumatoid arthritis can spread to the larger joints, including the hips and knees. Some will experience constitutional symptoms, such as loss of appetite, loss of weight, fever, and fatigue.

The pain of rheumatoid arthritis is generally more prominent in the early morning and gets somewhat better during the day. This is different from the pain of osteoarthritis, which tends to be less in the morning and gets worse during the day.

How is rheumatoid arthritis treated?

As with any form of arthritis, cooperation between the patient and the physician is very important. Overall, the treatment for rheumatoid arthritis is similar in approach to that for osteoarthritis—the relief of pain, the appropriate exercise and rest, and medication. Your physician will map out a plan combining these 3 components of treatment. It is imperative that you follow his or her directions to the letter.

Rheumatoid arthritis usually responds very well to treatment but often takes a long period of time before the patient begins to feel any relief from the symptoms. The medications used to combat rheumatoid arthritis relieve the inflammation in the synovial lining and in the joint itself and thus curtail the destruction of the joint. However, there is some difference between the medicine used with rheumatoid arthritis and that used with osteoarthritis. Of course, anti-inflammatory medications are important, but with rheumatoid arthritis, there may be some help available through more sophisticated yet potentially dangerous

197

drugs. Some patients with severe rheumatoid arthritis have responded to medications once used only to treat malaria and/or cancer. Under the proper supervision of a physician, and given in proper doses, these medications can significantly reduce the pain of rheumatoid arthritis—as a last resort.

Another treatment for rheumatoid arthritis rarely used with osteoarthritis is the use of splints to relieve the pain. These splints immobilize certain joints and put them at rest. Immobilization of the joint in combination with heat, medications, and exercise can allow it to heal much faster.

If I have rheumatoid arthritis, what does my future hold?

It is impossible for your doctor to look into a crystal ball and tell you how far your rheumatoid arthritis will progress. The only thing we know for sure is that people with rheumatoid arthritis experience frequent remissions, but disease usually progresses. This progression will be manifested by continued destruction of certain joints, especially in the hands and feet.

Rheumatoid arthritis is also called deforming arthritis because it makes the joints of the fingers, hands, and feet become deformed and turn outward. This sort of deformity is much more rare in people with osteoarthritis. But again, through the proper use of a specially tailored treatment program using heat, medications, exercise, and splints, the occurrence of these deformities can be reduced.

GOUT

What is gout?

Gout is 1 of the oldest forms of inflammation of the joints known. People with gout have been noted throughout history. Remember the pictures of Benjamin Franklin sitting with his foot propped up on a cushion and wrapped in bandages? That's because Ben Franklin had gout.

Gout, the only form of arthritis definitely known to be inherited, results from an increase in uric acid in the blood system. This acid builds up because of an inherited tendency to produce too much uric acid or not get rid of it through urination. When the blood level of uric acid rises, the acid occasionally settles in joints throughout the body, causing acute inflammation and swelling.

About 800,000 people in the United States have gout; 95% of them are male. Gout can strike at any age, but it more commonly occurs between the ages of 30 and 50.

Why is all that excessive uric acid harmful?

Each of us produces uric acid every day, but it is generally discharged from the body through the urine and doesn't have time to build up. If a person produces too much uric acid or cannot eliminate enough, the level in the blood becomes too high. Since the acid doesn't dissolve in the body fluids, it forms crystals, called tophi, that precipitate out of the blood and settle in the joints. Most often these deposits occur around the big toe, but they can also affect other areas, such as the feet, the hands, the lower back, and, occasionally, the ear. When these crystals form, they cause a great deal of inflammation in the joint lining, producing swelling, redness, and pain.

I've heard that only the rich get gout.

The myth that gout affects only the rich came about because historically, the people who could afford red meat and alcohol, which tend to increase the amount of uric acid produced, were the rich. Gout became known as a rich man's disease. Actually, people of all ages and socioeconomic backgrounds suffer from gout. The key is whether or not a tendency for gout runs in your family.

What are some of the symptoms of an acute attack of gout?

People with gout have a constant elevation of their uric acid level, but there is a point when the acid crystals lodge in the joint and cause a sudden and severe 1st attack. The big joint of the big toe is the primary location of the 1st attack of gout in 50% to 75% of people. Other frequent sites of the 1st attack are the knee, ankle, hand, wrist, and elbow joints. The hips and shoulders are rarely affected.

As noted, the pain of gout is caused by the inflammation reaction set off when the uric acid crystals form in the joint. As cells are destroyed because of the inflammation, they release enzymes and other chemicals that prolong the pain, swelling, and redness. Unlike other kinds of arthritis, gout attacks begin suddenly, often with a searing pain severe enough to awaken someone out of a sound sleep.

What triggers the 1st attack of gout?

The answer to this question is different with each individual. For some people, a severe emotional upset can cause an attack. Others may have an attack after having a particular type of food or drink. An injury such as a fall or a twisted knee, can trigger an attack, as can a change in the weather or the use of certain drugs. But most often, there are no discernible reasons or universal rules to explain what triggers the 1st attack of gout.

199

How is gout treated?

The primary treatment for gout is to keep a normal level of uric acid in the blood, and 2 medications are available to do this. These drugs, introduced in the early 1960s, have changed gout from a disastrously crippling disease to a relatively minor inconvenience.

These drugs reduce the uric acid level in the blood in 2 ways. The medication probenecid helps the kidneys excrete more of the uric acid. The newest gout drug, allopurinol, reduces the amount of uric acid the body manufactures. For most people, these medications significantly lower the uric acid level in the blood.

Antigout medicines *must* be taken as prescribed by your doctor. If given at the wrong times or in incorrect amounts, they may be ineffective and may cause unpleasant side effects. How and when you take the medication will depend on your particular case. If your gout is severe, you may need to take the medication for the rest of your life. On the other hand, you may need to take the medication only long enough to bring the acid level under control.

An acute attack of gout is treated somewhat differently. A medication called colchicine is given every hour for up to 6 hours or until diarrhea occurs. Colchicine combined with pain-reducing and anti-inflammatory medicines can significantly reduce the sudden pain from acute gout.

What role does diet play in gout?

The uric acid in the system comes from chemicals called purines that the body manufactures from raw materials or absorbs from foods. A simple measure that can help keep uric acid levels low is to eat a diet that does not contain purine-rich foods. Foods very high in purine content are all of the organ meats (brains, liver, kidney, sweetbreads), anchovies, salmon, perch, and sardines. Foods fairly high in purine content are asparagus, beans, fish, mushrooms, onions, oatmeal, peppers, and poultry.

OTHER TYPES OF ARTHRITIS

What are some other types of arthritis?

The 3 kinds of arthritis discussed here cover over 90% of the patients in this country, but there are other types. I can mention only a few.

Many people have heard of the disease lupus, but few know that it is associated with a particular form of arthritis. Thyroid disease, especially low thyroid (hypothyroidism), can also be associated with a form of arthritis. Psoriasis, in its most severe form, has a particular condition called psoriatic arthritis. Some unusual forms of arthritis are associated with inflammatory bowel diseases and with bacterial, viral, and gonorrheal infections.

LUPUS

What is lupus?

Lupus or, more correctly, lupus erythematosus is an example of a group of different problems referred to as immune complex diseases. Through complex mechanisms, the normal defense systems of the lupus patient are altered, damaging healthy tissue. To date, we are not sure why this occurs, but when it does, it can have serious consequences.

The onset of lupus is most common in females between the ages of 9 and 15 years. It can, however, manifest itself any time throughout adulthood. Lupus can affect any part of the body, from the joints and muscles to the liver, kidney, and brain. By far, the most common site is the joints.

A lupus patient often has a "butterfly" rash appearing on the cheeks. An extreme sensitivity to the sun is also common.

The treatment of lupus depends on which part of the body is affected. Advanced methods of treating this disease, once thought to be deadly, have greatly improved the chances of a lupus patient's living a productive life.

BURSITIS

What is bursitis?

In your body, wherever muscles and bones come together is a small, fluid-filled sac that provides padding and lubrication—the bursa. Bursitis is an inflammation of this sac, and most commonly involves the shoulder, elbow, wrist, hip, knee, or ankle.

Bursitis results from an overuse of a particular joint. Chopping a lot of wood may cause shoulder bursitis; carpenters or other workers who constantly crawl around on their knees may suffer from housemaid's knee. A person with bursitis has pain when moving the joint, but the joint *can* be freely moved. Pressing on the bursa from the outside causes pain, and there may also be some degree of redness, swelling, or warmth.

How do you treat bursitis?

201

The most important factor in the treatment of bursitis is to make sure that's what you have. Other causes of painful joints must be ruled out. An individual who complains of pain with movement of a joint and has localized tenderness but can move the joint well probably has bursitis.

The next thing to do is to put that particular joint to rest. If you've gotten bursitis of the shoulder from chopping wood and you continue to chop wood, your shoulder won't get any better. Stop the offending activity, then treat the bursa with applications of heat by using heating pads or hot towels or by standing under a hot shower. Do this for approximately 30 minutes, 3 to 4 times a day.

Your physician will probably want to place you on aspirin or a nonsteroidal anti-inflammatory drug to relieve the pain and the inflammation of the sac while your body's natural healing process continues.

If your bursitis does not respond to these simple measures, your physician may recommend that you have an injection of cortisone. Cortisone is an ultimate drug for the control of inflammation. It has potential side effects, but when given in an injection into 1 joint, it causes few problems.

How can I avoid future problems with bursitis?

The best way to prevent future attacks of bursitis is to strengthen the muscles around the joint and keep the joint limber. This can be accomplished by using exercises specially tailored for the joint with the inflammation. These exercises, if done properly, can strengthen the joint enough so that you can return to the activity that precipitated the original attack without fear of future bouts of bursitis.

TENDONITIS

What is tendonitis?

Tendonitis is inflammation of the tendon, the strong fibrous tissue that connects a muscle to a bone. When these tendons are stretched beyond their normal range or are overused, they can become inflamed. The symptoms of tendonitis are the same as any other inflammatory process—pain, swelling, redness, and warmth. The tendons most commonly affected are those of the wrist, forearm, knee, hand, and lower leg.

Let's look at a fairly common story. A man does a lot of yard work and chops down a few trees over the weekend. He feels fine while he is doing all this, but 12 or more hours later, he develops severe pain in his wrist. The pain gets worse when he rotates the wrist and is especially bad when he tries to grip or pull on anything. There is localized tenderness, redness, and warmth in the wrist area, although the wrist joint itself can be moved. A person who experiences this type of symptom—no matter where it occurs in the body—probably has tendonitis.

How do you treat tendonitis?

The treatment of all inflammatory processes is basically the same. Put the affected part at rest, apply heat, and take anti-inflammatory medications. These are very simple things that you can do at home for 2 or 3 days. If taking 2 aspirin, 4 times a day with meals or milk, and the applying of heat for 30 minutes, 3 or 4 times a day, do not significantly reduce your symptoms, you should consult your physician.

MYOSITIS

What is myositis?

Myositis is an inflammation of your muscles. As in bursitis and tendonitis, the most common cause of myositis is overuse. People who suddenly undertake certain vigorous activities, such as jogging, running, or prolonged walking, may wake up the next morning with painfully swollen muscles. If your muscle is painful to the touch, is swollen, feels warm, or has some redness, you probably have an acute case of myositis.

Again, the treatment is to place the muscle at rest, apply hot packs and, if you can tolerate them, take aspirin for 2 to 3 days. After the pain has subsided and the swelling has gone away, you should be able to return to your normal routine.

Remember, however, that if you have had any of these forms of inflammation, you've done something to precipitate them. Review the activities that may have caused the problem, and avoid overdoing those activities in the future or at least make sure that you do strengthening exercises for the affected limb.

LOW BACK PAIN

What is low back pain?

Second only to the common cold, low back pain is the most common cause of disability and work absences. Walking upright puts a lot of stress and strain on the lower back.

The backbone, or spinal column is a series of 24 separate vertebrae (bones shaped like boxes) stacked on top of each other. The lower section of the spine is composed of the sacrum and the coccyx, which are in reality fused vertebrae. These bones are supported by firm muscles that run on either side from the base of the head and neck to the lower portion of the buttocks. It is relatively common for people, especially those who are out of shape, to pull or acutely strain the muscles of the lower back.

Almost all of us, at some time or another, have tried to lift a box or piece of furniture that was too heavy and then suffered a rather severe pain in the lower back. Many times, this pain will go away if we simply apply some heat and rest for a few hours. At other times, however, the pain is so intense that it is almost impossible to move. When this happens, you have suffered an acute strain of your lower back muscles, or lumbosacral strain.

The best therapy is to immediately get off your feet and into bed. A firm mattress or even the floor is most comfortable. You should move only to go to the bathroom and to eat. While you rest, apply heat to your lower back with a heating pad or hot-water bottle, but only for 30 to 45 minutes, 4 to 5 times a day. Aspirin can relieve some of the discomfort, but if the pain continues more than 24 hours, you will probably need a muscle relaxant or an anti-inflammatory medication from your physician.

If the pain does not go away or if you develop numbness, tingling, or weakness in your leg or foot, consult your physician. You may have done more than simply strained a muscle.

What is a ruptured disk?

Your backbone, or spine, is made up of individual bones (vertebrae) that protect the nerves of the spinal column from injury. Each vertebra is separated by a cushion called a disk. The function of the disk is to keep the bones of the spine from rubbing together.

From special openings between these vertebrae, the nerve of the spinal column sends individual nerves to all parts of the body. In the lower back, the nerves that control the legs leave the spinal column between each low back, or lumbar, vertebra.

The nerves travel along smooth, open pathways as long as the cushions, disks, are keeping the vertebrae apart. However, during certain injuries or when straining your back, a disk can rupture through the protective capsule and cause the nerve to be pinched by either the displaced disk or the vertebra. When this occurs, the irritated nerve will send pain, numbness, tingling, and sometimes weakness down the leg. This is referred to as a ruptured disk and many times requires surgical treatment.

15.

Sports Medicine

PHYSICAL EXAM

Should an individual have a physical exam before active participation in a sport?

Anyone who is about to begin active participation in a sport should have a thorough evaluation by a physician. This applies especially to children and teenagers but goes for adults, too.

The 1st reason a physical examination is important is to assess the overall health of the athlete. During this evaluation, the physician will make sure that the individual's heart, lungs, blood pressure, and general condition are sound. He or she will also perform some laboratory analyses to make sure there is no underlying diabetes or anemia that could contribute to poor performance or possible injury.

The 2nd reason for this evaluation is to uncover any specific problem that could predispose someone to injury. The physician will pay particular attention to the skeletal and muscle system and will evaluate the bones, joints, and muscle strength throughout the body to make sure that there is no particular tightness or laxity that could contribute to injuries. For example, if the physician finds that the person's knee ligaments are particularly loose, providing proper knee support and exercises could prevent a crippling injury.

A 3rd reason to have a medical evaluation prior to participation in sports is to help the athlete determine an optimum level of performance. Unrealistic expectations during participation in sports are the leading causes of injury and frustration. With the help of a thorough evaluation, the physician and patient can sit down and try to determine the limits the patient should heed.

Following these guidelines will contribute to the overall health of the athlete and will help the athlete achieve the maximum benefit from any chosen sport.

DIET

Should athletes who participate regularly in a sport follow a special diet?

It is important for all of us to maintain a well-balanced diet. The athlete is no exception and should eat well-balanced meals that will supply the essential calories, vitamins, minerals, and nutrients for proper energy and maintenance of strength. There are always "fad" diets for athletes to follow, but sporting experts around the country agree that the best way to maintain proper performance is to follow a well-balanced diet.

A well-balanced diet includes selections *each day* from all 4 basic food groups. As we discussed in an earlier chapter, each group provides certain nutrients that are essential for proper energy and muscle function. For the athlete it is important to eat complex carbohydrates, foods such as potatoes, rice, pasta, beans, and corn. Because they provide essential fiber and are excellent sources of energy, they should be included at almost every meal.

Although fats have more than twice the calories of either protein or carbohydrates, they are still essential for proper functioning. Foods containing the healthier polyunsaturated or vegetable fats should be included to boost calories. Good choices include margarine, peanut butter, soybeans, and unsaturated salad dressings. Avoid the excessive amounts of cholesterol found in fatty meats, whole milk, and ice cream.

Another important component to an athletic diet that provides essential support maintenance for muscle tissue is protein. The amount of protein required by an average-sized adult is approximately 65 grams a day and will allow the athlete to maintain current body mass and weight. Almost all of the basic food groups (except fruits) supply some protein and should be included in the normal daily balanced diet.

An athlete who follows these basic premises can maintain enough protein, fats, and caloric intake for proper conditioning, strengthening, and performance.

AVOIDING INJURY

What's the best way to avoid sporting injuries?

206

Many common sporting injuries could be avoided if athletes would simply pay attention to the basics: warm-up exercises. Stretching and limbering exercises, done regularly and correctly before athletic activity, can help keep the body "in tune" for strenuous exercise. When the body is in tune, it is much less vulnerable to muscle stress, undue fatigue, and injury.

Regardless of the sport you participate in, these simple exercises not only help prevent injury but also allow you to perform at your optimum level. Do the following exercises for approximately 5 to 10 minutes before *any* sporting activity.

Stretching exercises. Regardless of the shape you're in, when you begin your activity, your muscles are usually tight, and tight muscles are much more prone to injury. So, your 1st set of exercises needs to gently, but progressively, stretch the major muscles of your body. Start with calf-stretching exercises. You can do them by leaning against a wall with both hands and placing 1 leg behind you. To stretch your calf muscles, lean forward keeping 1 foot planted behind you. Begin very gradually, and with each repetition, lean forward more, further stretching your calf and Achilles tendon. Repeat with the other leg back.

Limbering exercises. Gently jogging in place can limber up the major muscles in your legs. You should jog for approximately 3 to 5 minutes, gradually lifting your knees a little higher.

Upper trunk exercises. Many athletes will warm and limber up their leg muscles but forget that the upper trunk is also tight. Lateral bending exercises to loosen the trunk muscles begin by spreading your feet approximately shoulder-width apart and bending sideways and forward from the waist 10 repetitions each way. Trunk twists will also help loosen up the muscles of the trunk and lower back. Twist (gently) to the left and the right, 10 times each way.

Back-stretching exercises. Almost all sporting activities place some degree of stress on your lower back. Because this is a very critical area for injury, you should stretch your back by doing alternate toe-touching exercises. Again, placing your legs shoulder-width apart, reach down and touch your right foot with your left hand, come back up, then touch your left foot with your right hand. Touch each foot 10 times.

Remember that stretching exercises do the most good if done slowly and smoothly. Jerking the muscles or forcing them to stretch more than they can will only make them tighter and may cause injury.

How important is the "cool down"?

If you have ever gone to a horse race, you've seen that the owners and trainers pay close attention to the horses after the race. No horse is brought directly in from the race to the stall. Instead, they place a blanket over the horse to prevent it from cooling down too rapidly, and then they walk it for several minutes to let it cool down. Horse trainers have known for years that this prevents many injuries in subsequent workouts and races.

This cool-down period is equally important for any athlete. A common mistake made by joggers is to run their distance, then immediately go inside and sit down. When you finish your exercise, your muscles are extremely loose, but they will tighten too quickly if you don't have a cool-down period. Instead of immediately stopping all exercises, walk or jog gently for approximately 3 to 5 minutes after you finish your workout. Shake your arms and legs, extend your arms, and rotate them forward and back several times. Rotate your neck and shoulders to allow the muscles to cool off gradually and firm up. You should also avoid any extremes in temperature. Running in the hot summer sun and then immediately going into an air-conditioned house can contribute to increased muscle injuries.

What else can I do to keep from injuring myself?

Injuries are what people participating in sports fear the most. Besides being in good physical health, knowing the limits to which you can push yourself, and remembering the importance of warm-up exercises and cool-down periods, you can follow 3 more rules to prevent possible injury.

1. Don't overdo. The number 1 cause of injuries in the nonprofessional athlete is pushing too much. People simply try to accomplish things that they should not be trying to accomplish. Listen to your body. When your body feels that you are reaching your limits in a particular activity, it will tell you. You may develop unusual fatigue, some muscle soreness, or perhaps a pain that you are not used to having. Any of these can be potential signs of pushing yourself beyond safe limits.

2. Exercise in the right place. A recent study in North Carolina found that many of the injuries received in football programs were directly related to the playing conditions. Improving the conditions of the field dramatically reduced the number of injuries. We can all learn a great deal from this, no matter what the exercise or athletic competition. More than 1 jogger has sustained a significant injury by trying to jog on uneven surfaces or at night on unfamiliar terrain.

3. Use the proper equipment. Wear the proper shoes for your sport, and use the proper protective gear. Putting on a pair of goggles while playing racquetball will reduce the chance of serious eye injuries. Making sure your bike is the right size and properly maintained will make for a safer ride. The proper protective gear in any sport is critical for the prevention of significant injuries.

MUSCLE SORENESS

Why do my muscles feel so sore after I exercise?

Exercise of any nature can cause muscle soreness. The amount of soreness you have and when you experience it depend on the type of exercise you've been doing. There are basically 2 types of muscle soreness: the kind that occurs during exercise (acute muscle soreness), and the kind that occurs a day or 2 later (delayed muscle soreness).

Acute muscle soreness is associated with an inadequate blood supply that can happen during exercise. Many types of exercise, especially those involving resistance, actually reduce the flow of blood to the muscle and cause a buildup of by-products, including lactic acid. It is believed that the lactic acid stimulates the nerves and creates pain. Acute muscle soreness will fade relatively quickly after the exercise is stopped.

Delayed muscle soreness comes from actual damage to the muscle itself. When strenuous exercise damages the individual muscle fibers, these fibers swell, stimulating some of the sensitive nerve endings and creating soreness. The treatment of delayed muscle soreness includes massage, heat, and rest. Normally, this type of soreness is self-limiting and will go away in 2 or 3 days.

It is generally assumed that once muscles are in shape, soreness will not occur. This is not entirely so. Extreme acceleration of your training program can result in muscle soreness, even if you exercise regularly.

WEEKEND ATHLETE

I exercise only on weekends. Is that still beneficial for me?

A common excuse for not exercising regularly is "I'm too busy." In our fast-paced society, this is probably true for most individuals; unfortunately, weekend exercise programs are probably not totally adequate to maintain maximum benefits. In fact, the "weekend warrior" suffers more from muscle soreness, swollen joints, bruising, and more serious injuries than the person who works out regularly. Of course, it helps a great deal emotionally to exercise on the weekend, but everyone should make a special effort to extend that exercise program to 2 or 3 times during the week.

SPRAIN OR STRAIN?

What's the difference between a sprain and a strain?

It has been estimated that sprains and strains account for over 76% of all athletic injuries. The novice athlete considers them a minor nuisance, but professionals know that these 2 conditions can be serious and, if improperly treated, can lead to disability.

A sprain is an injury to the ligaments that surround the joint. In a sprain, the ligament fibers have been stretched beyond their limitations. In severe sprains, these fibers can be partially or totally torn.

A strain, on the other hand, is an injury to the muscle, the tendon, or the junction where the muscle and the tendon meet. Strains are often associated with muscle contraction and/or stretching of this muscle-tendon unit and are seldom associated with direct trauma or blow to the muscle.

Ice or heat?

A long-standing controversy is whether to treat acute strains or sprains with ice or heat. Time and time again, athletes sprain an ankle or strain a calf muscle and immediately apply heat; then they show up at the physician's office the next day or so, complaining of severe swelling.

Whether you're dealing with a sprain or a strain, there has been injury to tissue, often accompanied by some degree of bleeding and increased tissue fluid. Heat will actually stimulate blood supply to this area and increase the possibility of dramatic swelling.

Ice, on the other hand, not only provides an anesthetic response but temporarily reduces the blood supply to the area. Thus, it can prevent a significant amount of swelling.

Because the recovery period is lengthened when there has been excessive swelling, it is critical that ice packs be applied immediately to any sprain or strain.

RUNNING OR JOGGING SAFELY

How can I select the best running shoe for me?

To give yourself the maximum balance, strength, stability, comfort, and performance, you must select the proper footwear. Proper footwear not only increases your performance but significantly reduces your chances of developing leg and foot injuries. Here are some points to consider when selecting your shoes:
• Make sure that your shoe has a good heel counter to prevent pronation—the rolling of the foot that can cause stress fractures and runner's knee.

- There should be a built-in heel wedge to relieve the strain on the Achilles tendon and prevent tendonitis or Achilles tendon pulls.
- Because the heel strike is so important in jogging, make sure that your heel has a rounded bevel to ease the stress.
- The shoes should have a good insole for arch support, a good midsole to cushion the foot and to prevent shinsplints, and a waffle-studded base to absorb the shock.
- The best shoe for you contains all of the qualities mentioned above, feels comfortable, and wears well.

If you jog regularly, when your shoes begin to lose their studded sole, flexibility, and/or comfort, you should get new ones. Frequent runners usually need a new pair of shoes about every 3 to 6 months.

What are shinsplints?

The term *shinsplints* has really been used as a catchall to describe almost all conditions involving the lower leg around the shin or the muscles of the middle part of the lower leg. In general, shinsplints are strains that occur where the muscles at the back of the calf attach to the larger bone of the lower leg, the tibia.

The occurrence of shinsplints are related to the surface you are running on, your shoes, or a rather sudden acceleration in the amount of running you do. With shinsplints, the throbbing pain is located deep inside the lower leg and becomes worse at night. Continued running makes the pain much worse.

Almost all conditions categorized as shinsplints are caused by an improper running style. Instead of running in a normal position, the person will generally run with the feet turned slightly inward, transferring a great portion of the stress to a small group of muscles on the inside of the lower leg.

The best treatment for shinsplints is to rest the leg for 3 to 5 days. To reduce the inflammation, place ice packs on the leg for 15 to 20 minutes, 3 or 4 times a day. Taking 2 aspirins with each meal can also help reduce inflammation.

However, even better than trying to treat shinsplints is to prevent them. Make sure that you have a stable shoe that gives you plenty of heel and sole support. You should also reevaluate the surface on which you run if the problem continues.

What causes "runner's knee"?

The basic structures surrounding the knee are prone to injury while jogging. Let's look at the basic structure. The front part of the upper leg, the quadriceps muscle, is attached to the knee by a series of ligaments. This thick, strong ligament, known as the iliotibial band, is located on the outside of the upper leg and supports the outside of the knee.

The kneecap is actually a floating bone supported by the lower tendon of the quadriceps muscle. This tendon covers the kneecap, holding it in place, and attaches at the upper portion of the lower leg below the knee. The patellar tendon stretches from the kneecap to the upper portion of the lower leg.

Jogging can create numerous knee problems. The kneecap itself is prone to an inflammation of the sac around the knee (plica syndrome) or an inflammation of the undersurface of the kneecap (chondromalacia). The stress created by jogging can also irritate and strain the iliotibial band or the patellar tendon. Any of these conditions that affect the knee area and are caused by jogging or other running exercises are lumped together as runner's knee. Now let's look at some specific problems in more detail.

My quadriceps muscle hurts after running. What should I do?

If you experience pain in your quadriceps muscle, especially on the lower outside of the muscle, you could have iliotibial tendonitis, an irritation or inflammation of the band on the outside of the knee. With this condition, prolonged running may cause pain, stiffness, and an inability to freely move the knee. If you are experiencing these symptoms, the 1st thing you should do is *not* jog for 2 or 3 days. During that time, apply ice massages to the area 3 or 4 times a day for 10 to 15 minutes at a time. You should also take 2 aspirin with each meal and 2 at bedtime with a glass of milk. After 3 or 4 days, if the tenderness and swelling are reduced, you may begin to jog again. Begin *very* slowly and avoid strenuous workouts, jogging up and down steep hills, and jogging on uneven surfaces.

A common cause of iliotibial tendonitis is an improperly fitting shoe. Reevaluate your shoe support, making sure that your shoes are the proper size and fit, that they have not lost their support, and that the soles are not worn.

What should I do if I have some stiffness in my knee after jogging?

Some stiffness in your knee after jogging could be a sign of an inflammation of the patella. You may find that the pain is a little worse when getting out of a chair or walking up and down stairs. You might even hear a slight popping or grinding sound as you walk up the steps.

All of these symptoms are fairly common signs of chondromalacia of the patella, an inflammation or irritation of the undersurface of the kneecap. The kneecap, remember, is supported by the tendons of the quadriceps muscle. If there is some looseness in the muscle or the tendons, the kneecap will glide unevenly and cause an irritation or inflammation of the undersurface.

An acute attack of chondromalacia is best treated by discontinuing jogging for about a week. Take 2 aspirin at each meal and at bedtime. Put ice packs right on top of the kneecap for 20 to 30 minutes, 3 or 4 times a day. When the tenderness and inflammation subside and you can do a light jog without the recurrence of pain, you can probably return to your jogging program, but at a much slower pace. The most common causes of chondromalacia are improperly fitting shoes and a weak quadriceps muscle. We've discussed the importance of properly fitting shoes, so now let's turn our attention to quadriceps-strengthening exercises.

How do you do quadriceps-strengthening exercises?

If your physician finds that your knee problems from jogging are related to weak quadriceps muscles, he or she will recommend special strengthening exercises to prevent the problems in the future. Basically the muscle should be tightly contracted, held for approximately 10 seconds, and then relaxed. To tighten the quadriceps muscle, simply extend your leg straight out and pull your toe back toward your head. Do that now, while you're reading. The large muscle on the top of your leg that tightens up is the quadriceps. Performing this stretching and pulling exercise 20 times, 4 to 5 times a day, will greatly increase the strength and the support of the quadriceps.

Another way to do quadriceps-strengthening exercises is to lift weights with the leg; a special quadriceps machine will enable you to do this. But remember, never try to lift too much weight. If you have weak quads, you should begin by lifting no more than 5 to 10 pounds with each leg, gradually bulding up to 25 to 30 pounds over several weeks. Exercises can be done in repetitions of 20.

However, you don't have to have a machine to accomplish the same thing. Take a large satchel or pocketbook that has big loop handles, place an empty 6-pack of soft drink bottles in the bottom, place the loops around your foot, and sit on the edge of a table or chair high enough so that you can dangle your legs. Then lift the satchel. Do this for 20 repetitions with each leg, 2 or 3 times a day. Approximately every week, replace an empty bottle with a full 1. Over the 6 weeks, you will be increasing the weight you're lifting from 4 or 5 pounds to 15 or 20. One should never begin these exercises without first consulting a physician.

THE KNEE

What if my knee pain continues, recurs, or the swelling doesn't go away?

Persistent knee pain, especially associated with swelling that will not resolve, must be evaluated by your physician. Constant pain and swelling could indicate a problem deep inside the knee structure itself, perhaps a tear of a ligament or some cartilage or a more significant injury. For many inflammations, it is appropriate for you to treat yourself as described. But if your knee is not well within a week, especially if the pain is associated with difficulty in walking, a giving way of the knee, or a locking of the knee so you can't move it for a few seconds, you should contact your physician for further evaluation.

How can I treat a sprained knee?

As we've discussed, the knee is prone to injury in athletic endeavors because the knee joint itself is supported by the muscles of the upper leg, the quadriceps, and ligaments extending on either side of the knee joint. If these ligaments or these muscles are not strong enough and if the joint itself has undue stress, then injury can occur.

A sprained knee means that the knee has been moved in an unnatural motion. It responds by a sudden onset of pain and swelling and an inability to walk properly.

Your immediate response should be to apply ice to the knee and get off your feet. The ice will help prevent any undue swelling within the knee joint itself. After 4 to 6 hours if your knee is feeling better and there is no undue swelling, try to do a little bit of walking, but do not return to your exercise. If the pain continues and if the swelling does not resolve within 24 to 48 hours, consult your physician to make sure there is no further damage in the knee.

What causes a torn ligament in the knee?

Most of us have seen a football game in which the runner is tackled from the side and he immediately goes down, holding his knee. What has happened is that while he is running, his cleats are planted firmly in the ground, taking away any ability of the knee to give on impact. At the same time, the runner is often twisting or turning the knee at the moment of impact. Since the knee simply cannot withstand that sort of stress, a ligament pops—a "torn" ligament.

The symptoms of a torn ligament are immediate pain and swelling. Although the knee can be moved, it is very unstable. If this has happened to you, immediately consult an orthopedist or sports medicine specialist for treatment. Torn ligaments on either side of the knee often have to be repaired surgically.

What's the difference between a torn ligament and torn cartilage?

The knee ligaments are the strong bands that support the knee. The cartilage, on the other hand, is the thick, fibrous tissue inside the knee joint that makes a cushion between the upper bone (the femur) and the lower 2 bones of the leg. Torn cartilage happens when a runner plants the cleated foot and then tries to twist to one side. The foot cannot twist, but the knee will, and the cartilage tears.

The symptoms of torn cartilage are sudden pains that will generally subside. The player may even get back up on the leg and run some more. However, in a few minutes, the knee will begin to swell, and the torn cartilage will lock the knee so it cannot be moved. Torn cartilage, like torn ligaments, needs evaluation by an orthopedic or sports medicine specialist. With the help of arthroscopy, actually looking into the knee joint with a small microscope, the correct diagnosis can be made and appropriate therapy instituted.

THE ANKLE

What exactly is a sprained ankle?

A sprained ankle is a frequent injury in almost any athletic event, but especially in tennis, basketball, football, and running. Sprained ankles are generally considered to be minor problems, but they are also a leading cause of disability in athletes. In the Winter Olympic Games in 1971, for example, 33% of all injuries were ankle injuries. It has been estimated that 1 out of every 4 ankle sprains results in recurrent disability.

To understand what causes a sprained ankle, you have to understand that the ankle itself is a joint, where the 2 bones of the lower leg (tibia and fibula) attach to the foot. The protruding "bone" of the lower leg that we generally refer to as the ankle is really the lower portion of the 2 bones. These bones are attached to the foot by a series of very strong, fibrous ligaments on the inside and the outside of the ankle.

215

A sprained ankle occurs when, for whatever reason, the ankle is forcefully turned in or out and undue strain is put on those ligaments. Ankle sprains can be minor or so severe that the ligament actually ruptures.

The symptoms of a sprained ankle are sudden onsets of swelling and pain and an inability to walk. If not treated, the swelling can progress to the point where you cannot put on your shoe.

What should I do if I have sprained my ankle?

Apply ice immediately. Swelling comes from a large amount of fluid that seeps out into the tissue in response to the injury. Bleeding can occur from actual rupturing of blood vessels under the skin and cause bruising and more swelling. To reduce the amount of swelling, immediately place ice on the ankle to temporarily reduce the amount of blood and fluid flowing to the area. If heat is applied, the swelling will get worse because the blood supply is increased. The next thing is to get off your foot and elevate it. The combination of ice packs and elevation can significantly reduce the swelling that greatly contributes to the pain and disability. An anti-inflammatory medication such as aspirin, taken 4 times a day, can reduce the discomfort.

How long should I stay off my sprained ankle?

You should stay off your ankle—and not apply any pressure or walk on it—until the swelling has totally subsided. Swelling in the ankle indicates that the ankle joint itself is still very weak. Until that swelling goes away, it's going to be very difficult for your ankle ligaments to support your weight. You may need to walk around on crutches for a while, depending on the severity of the sprain. After the swelling subsides, continue using the crutches, but apply more and more weight each day to the ankle until the pain and swelling subside entirely and you can walk normally.

Should I tape my ankles prior to exercising?

Although ankle injuries are extremely common in athletes, deciding whether or not to tape your ankles is difficult. Many professional athletes, notably football players, always tape their ankles before a game. However, I don't believe that this procedure applies to the average non-professional athlete.

Taping can prevent certain sports-related injuries; it can also create them if improperly done. Simply throwing an elastic bandage around your ankle is not adequate protection. If you have not suffered ankle injuries and if, during your evaluation by your physician, no looseness of the ankle joints is found, the best bet is to support your ankles with proper footwear, not with tape.

If you've had some injury to your ankles, then you have a choice: learn from a professional exactly how to tape your ankles, or use a slip-on elastic sock that can be purchased at a sporting goods store. This type of support has an opening for the toes and heel and fits snugly against the ankle. Wear it during the athletic event, but take it off at other times.

How can I prevent a sprained ankle?

If you know that you have "weak" ankles, or if you have been prone to sprained ankles in the past, there are some special exercises you can do to strengthen the ankle ligaments. For example, stand on your tip-toes for several minutes and then rock back, standing on your heels. After this, turn your ankle inward and outward approximately 20 times before beginning the exercise you're planning. Ankle supports from your local sporting goods store can help support the ankle but be cautious in using them unless they have been recommended by your physician. When outside supports are used, the normal ligaments of your ankle are less likely to firm up and get stronger.

STRESS FRACTURE

What are stress fractures?

Stress fractures are caused by repetitive force that causes damage over a period of time. People with stress fractures will have a rather characteristic history. The pain can be localized, can radiate to other parts of the foot, or can be felt only in a joint of the foot. When the pain occurs, no specific injury can be identified. The pain responds well to rest but will recur when exercise is resumed.

A history of running is a tip-off that a person could have a stress fracture. This type of fracture is odd because in most cases, normal x-rays are totally negative up to 3 weeks after the fracture occurs. Often, the fracture will not appear until it has begun to heal and forms a callus.

Early diagnosis of stress fractures is desirable but difficult. Sometimes special bone scan x-rays must be performed to find the specific fracture site.

Stress fractures are best treated by resting and by avoiding whatever caused the injury. Runners should curtail their running for 4 to 6 weeks

217

or until the fracture totally heals. Rehabilitation is a major part of the healing process and must proceed very slowly.

THE HEEL

My heel hurts after exercising. What could be causing the pain?

Heel pain that occurs during and immediately after exercise could either be an indication of a bone bruise (a bruising of the heel bone) or a heel spur (a calcium deposit at the base of the heel). By far, however, the most common cause of this pain is plantar fascitis, an inflammation of the tissue in the sole of the foot where it attaches to the heel.

The diagnosis is generally made by checking the location of the pain by direct compression and by evaluating a history of running, lots of tennis, or other exercises that could put stress on the heel. Treatment includes rest, with a long period away from running or other aggravating exercises to allow the inflammation to subside. As with the treatment of other inflammations, heat and aspirin or anti-inflammatory medications are helpful.

The best way to prevent plantar fascitis is to select proper shoes that protect the heel.

TENNIS INJURIES

What causes tennis elbow?

Tennis elbow is, of course, a problem for tennis players, but golfers, carpenters, and baseball players get it, too. The phrase can be applied to any ongoing discomfort in the elbow.

The exact diagnosis of tennis elbow is epicondylitis, inflammation of the tendon that attaches the muscle of the forearm to the bone of the upper arm at the elbow. The classic symptom of tennis elbow is pain on the outside or inside of the elbow that gets worse upon gripping or twisting. There may also be other signs of inflammation, such as redness, swelling, and warmth.

Epicondylitis usually responds well to stopping the activity that creates the pain and letting the extremity rest. If possible, you *don't* want to place the arm in a sling, because this can lead to a weakening of the supporting muscles around the elbow.

If the condition has been present for several weeks, applying heat for 30 minutes 3 or 4 times a day will help, as will taking 2 aspirin 4 times a day with meals or milk. If the condition has persisted for some time, your physician may prescribe anti-inflammatory medications.

If the elbow does not respond to these measures, your physician may elect to try an injection of cortisone around the inflammation to reduce the pain.

Healing is complete when you have no residual pain as you resume your activities. Remember, as with other injuries, to take it slow.

How can I avoid tennis elbow?

The most common cause of tennis elbow is playing tennis with an improperly executed backhand, called the leading elbow stroke. At impact, the shoulder is elevated and the elbow points at the net, causing overextension and a snapping twist of the elbow. Prevention may be as simple as modifying the tension on the strings of your racquet or reverting to a 2-handed backhand. If that doesn't work, wrapping the forearm approximately 4" below the elbow, a counterforce brace, can reduce the muscular overload.

Every time I hit an overhead in tennis, I have pain in my shoulder.

The serve and the overhead in tennis are the main culprits in inflammations of the shoulder. This inflammation and the resulting pain can occur in any age group and at all levels of tennis play.

Watch someone serve powerfully or hit a strong overhead, and you can see the force and strain that are placed on the shoulder area. This overhead motion causes an impingement in the area where the muscles of the upper arm attach to the shoulder. People who have inflammation will aggravate the pain if they stand straight and try to elevate the arm outward above the level of their shoulder or make circular motions with the arm.

Chronic irritation can lead to an inflammatory process of the tendon called tendonitis. Repeated trauma can cause small tears that can lead to a breakdown of the shoulder joint. At this point, surgery is often required.

Treatment of the otherwise healthy athlete with shoulder pain is immediately icing the shoulder for at least 10 minutes after each workout. To decrease the inflammation, anti-inflammatory drugs may be prescribed. Aspirin is the least expensive anti-inflammatory drug and may be tried 1st.

If these simple measures do not reduce the pain, stop the aggravating activity and get a thorough physical examination to make sure there is no permanent damage to the muscle and tendons of the shoulder.

GOLFER'S BACK

When I play a lot of golf, my back hurts.

Have you ever watched your golf partner tee off? Next time, notice the tremendous exertion placed on the lower back. You're not only bending over, you're twisting your back rapidly from side to side and to a rather extreme degree. This makes the lower portion of the back prone to injury.

Another reason the lower back gives players trouble is that they do not pay adequate attention to warm-up exercises. So, prior to teeing off, spend 15 to 20 minutes doing range-of-motion exercises. Start warming up by gently twisting your torso from side to side, with your feet planted, arching your back backward, then forward about 45°. Another good, nonstressful exercise is to sit on the ground and bring your knees up to your chest 10 to 15 times.

The problems associated with playing golf, such as prolonged periods between each shot, predispose golfers to losing the benefits of the warm-up. So, if the weather is chilly or cold and if there's a wait between shots, repeat these warm-up exercises several times during the round.

If I have "golfer's back," how do I treat myself?

Golfer's back is caused by an inflammation of the muscles of the lower portion of the spine. These muscles have been stretched past their limits and are inflamed and tender. If the muscles are achy, but you can move your back in any direction without severe pain, the only treatment you may need is to get off your feet for a few hours, apply heat, and take some aspirin for a day or 2.

If, however, your back muscles are so inflamed and tightened that any movement of your back causes more pain, the best recommendation for you is strict bed rest—lying flat in bed, getting up only to eat and go to the bathroom. Apply heat or a heating pad to the lower back for 30 to 45 minutes every 2 to 3 hours. Note that it is better to put the heat on for a while and then take it off, allowing your back to cool, than it is to leave the heating pad on at all times.

If the pain does not subside within 24 to 48 hours, consult your physician. He or she will make sure you do not have a more serious injury and can prescribe medication to ease the inflammation.

16.

Problems of the Nervous System

STROKE

What is a stroke?

A stroke occurs when the blood supply to a portion of the brain is dramatically reduced or entirely shut off. As a result, the nerve cells in the portion of the brain nourished by that blood cannot function. When this occurs, the part of the body controlled by those nerve cells also cannot function. Results of the stroke may be weakness, a loss of feeling or paralysis of 1 side of the body, vision problems, inability to walk, or difficulty in speaking or understanding. These effects may be slight or severe; they may also be temporary or permanent.

How do strokes occur?

All strokes are an interference with the blood supply to a portion of the brain, but they can occur for many reasons. A clot may form in an artery of the brain and actually block the flow of blood to the brain tissue. This happens in arteries previously damaged by arterio-sclerosis—hardening of the arteries. Strokes may be cause by a hemor-rhage or bleeding from an artery that results when a diseased artery leaks or bursts and damages the surrounding brain tissue.

Strokes can also be caused when a blood clot, or embolus, breaks loose from the inner lining of the wall of the heart or a major artery leading to the brain, is carried to the brain, and blocks off a small artery.

Why do some people with strokes suffer only mild problems, while others are severely affected?

The extent of damage from a stroke will depend upon how large the clot or hemorrhage is and which of the arteries is totally blocked off. If a very small artery is blocked off only in the portion of the brain that controls the ability to speak properly, the effects of the stroke may be only slurring of the speech or the inability to speak clearly. However, if a large artery that supplies the portion of the brain that controls 1 whole side is blocked off, then that whole side of the body will cease functioning normally and the individual may be paralyzed.

Can the body ever repair itself after it has been damaged by a stroke?

Whenever the blood supply to a particular part of the body shuts off, the body immediately attempts to repair itself. Small blood vessels in the area of the blockage get larger in an attempt to take over the work of those damaged. If this happens after a stroke, some of the damaged nerve cells may be able to receive blood from these newer arteries and thus regain a portion of their normal function.

Some people begin to recover relatively quickly from a stroke, which means that the body's ability to replace the blood supply has been optimal. Those suffering more serious damage will take a longer time, if they can get enough blood supply from normal arteries to the damaged area. For others, however, the damage will be too severe for the body to repair itself, and they will not regain normal function.

How can I keep from having a stroke?

Regular medical checkups are probably the best way to prevent strokes. With the help of a comprehensive medical examination, your physician will be able to determine if you have any of the risk factors such as hypertension (high blood pressure), diabetes, diseases of the coronary arteries, or certain other heart or blood vessel diseases.

Control of high blood pressure or diabetes can dramatically decrease your chances of having a stroke in the future.

Finding narrowed arteries in the circulatory system, even though they have not caused any problems yet, may lead your physician to recommend surgery to open up arteries in the neck that are beginning to close. Correction of blockage in the neck arteries could prevent you from having a major stroke.

Medications that thin the blood—anticoagulants—may also be prescribed for some people to avert a 1st stroke or to prevent a 2nd.

If you have some of the risk factors, a physician will try to alleviate them by advising you to change certain health habits. Losing weight, lowering blood cholesterol levels, exercising moderately, and getting relief from stress can help you *not* have a stroke. Also, cigarette smoking is associated with an increased risk of strokes as well as heart attacks.

How are strokes treated once they occur?

Early and thorough diagnosis is of great urgency. As soon as possible, a physician will make a fairly definite diagnosis about what kind of stroke has occurred so that prompt medical or surgical treatment can be implemented.

But even with the great advances we have made in medical science, once a massive stroke has occurred, there is really very little that a physician can do. Many times physicians give the patient a type of medication that can help thin the blood. This medication (low molecular dextran) can, in some cases, increase the blood supply to the damaged area and thus facilitate some degree of recovery. It must be emphasized that in no way is this a guaranteed cure for a stroke; it is done to give the patient every benefit of increased circulation to the damaged area and, it is hoped, some degree of repair.

However, major advances have taken place in the successful rehabilitation of patients. Once the patient has been seen by a physician, regardless of the area where the stroke occurred, a rehabilitative program will be undertaken. This program uses a team approach to get the patient back to being as independent as possible as quickly as possible. Physical therapists deal with the physical aspects of the stroke, such as paralysis; speech therapists assist with the patient's inability to speak; and occupational therapists try to help patients regain self-sufficiency in normal activities of daily living. With the help of this special team, patients who suffer massive strokes, even though there is no cure, can regain the maximum possible level of functioning.

Can taking aspirin reduce my chances of having a serious stroke?

Studies show that taking small amounts of aspirin (1 baby aspirin tablet once a day) does have some effect on the ability of your blood to clot. Aspirin produces this thinning by decreasing the stickiness of the platelets in your blood. If you are in a high-risk category, your physician may recommend this approach.

What is a transient stroke?

223

Transient ischemic attacks, or TIA's, are brief episodes that can herald the onset of a major stroke. These episodes generally last only 5 to 10 minutes but occasionally as long as 24 hours. Individuals may have a sudden difficulty with speech, such as slurring or garbling of words. Other symptoms can be a rather dramatic visual problem that comes on without warning but clears up in a short time. More often, people have paralysis or extreme weakness on 1 side of the body, often affecting only 1 arm or 1 leg.

All of these symptoms come on rather quickly and leave almost as suddenly. If, for instance, you had extreme weakness so that you could not use your right arm for several minutes, then normal functioning came back after a short time, you could have experienced a transient ischemic attack or a "ministroke." The importance of identifying these symptoms is that they generally are warning signs of a true stroke.

What can be done for transient ischemic attacks?

If you are having transient ischemic attacks, your physician will immediately begin an evaluation to see if you have any of the risk factors for major strokes such as high blood pressure, elevated blood sugar, or major artery disease. Each risk factor needs to be thoroughly evaluated and, if possible, brought under control.

In many cases, people with transient ischemic attacks have narrowed areas in the carotid artery, the major artery in the neck that carries blood to the brain. If these areas of narrowing are found, your physician may recommend surgery to replace the carotid narrowing with a new portion of artery. This may dramatically reduce your chances of having a clot or piece of that damaged artery break off, carry itself into the brain tissue, and produce a major stroke.

People suffering from transient ischemic attacks may also benefit from taking medications that can produce some degree of blood thinning. Acetylsalicylic acid (aspirin) may help persons who are suffering from TIA's.

If you have had symptoms that could be related to a TIA, you should consult your physician immediately.

DIZZINESS AND VERTIGO

What is the difference between simple dizziness and vertigo?

To many people, *dizziness* and *vertigo* mean the same thing. However, we need to find some way to distinguish between these 2 sensations. If you go to your physician and complain of dizziness, his or her

224

1st task will be to discover whether you are suffering from dizziness or true vertigo. This is important because the causes of these 2 conditions are often entirely different, so the treatment would be different, also.

The term *dizziness* should be used to describe a feeling of light-headedness, unsteadiness, confusion, or a fainting feeling.

The term *vertigo* should be reserved to describe a sensation of motion. People with true vertigo feel as if they are stationary and objects are moving around them, or as if they are moving even when they are not.

What are some causes of dizziness?

Finding the cause of a patient's dizziness is often a frustrating task for a physician. The symptom of dizziness generally means that there is a disorder of at least 1 of 3 different body components: the visual pathways (a problem with the eyes), the inner ear mechanism, or the sensory tract of the central nervous system. Your orientation and balance can be maintained only if all 3 components function in unison. Disruption of 1 or more of these areas will cause you to have a sensation of dizziness.

A common cause of dizziness, especially in elderly people, is related to circulatory problems. When arteriosclerosis (hardening of the arteries) begins to affect the arteries of the brain, a person may experience difficulties with the inner ear mechanism due to lack of an adequate blood supply. This may be manifested as a ringing in the ear (tinnitus) or by a sensation of constant dizziness.

Many people with high blood pressure also complain of dizziness. Sometimes this dizziness occurs only when they stand up or change positions rather quickly; at other times they may experience it in waves.

Some other causes of dizziness are low blood pressure, anemia, hypothyroidism, and low blood sugar. If you experience constant dizziness that is interrupting your ability to lead a normal life, you should consult your physician. He or she will then have the task of making sure you are having dizziness and not vertigo, then trying to decide what causes it. Many of these causes are controllable, such as high blood pressure, hypothyroidism, or anemia. Others, such as hardening of the arteries, may not be correctable, and your physician will need to recommend treatment to enable you to cope with the symptoms.

What are some of the treatments for constant dizziness?

If your physician has determined that you suffer from a noncorrectable cause of dizziness, he or she will then recommend certain treatments to control the symptoms. Some dizziness may be controlled by

225

simply not changing positions too quickly. For example, do not bend down to tie your shoes, and then stand up immediately, or do not try to "hop" out of bed without 1st sitting on the side of the bed for a few minutes.

For some people, correcting dizziness may not be so simple, and a physician may need to prescribe medications that can help control the symptoms.

What are some of the causes of true vertigo?

True vertigo is a devastating problem to people who suffer from it constantly. True vertigo can be caused by a disruption of the inner ear mechanism, the eye mechanism, or the central nervous system. It is essential to find what causes the symptoms, because only then can adequate treatment be given.

Some of the more common causes of true vertigo are related to the hearing mechanism. Diseases that are associated with vertigo and a hearing loss include Ménière's disease, an inflammation of the inner ear mechanism called labyrinthitis and, very rarely, tumors of the brain that can cause a malfunction of the major nerve controlling the balance system.

Other causes of vertigo not associated with hearing loss include a relatively common condition known as benign positional vertigo and vestibular neuronitis, an inflammation of the nerve to the inner ear.

Problems with the blood vessels can also cause vertigo. People who suffer from strokes or transient ischemic attacks often have intermittent vertigo. In these cases, it is important to decide if the vascular system is causing the vertigo, because it could be a warning sign of major problems with the circulatory system of the brain.

Some of the other causes of vertigo are a decreased output of thyroid hormone, low blood sugar, high blood pressure, low blood pressure, and anemia.

What are some of the treatments of true vertigo?

If your physician finds that your vertigo is triggered by problems with your inner ear, he or she will try to make sure that you don't have a tumor (acoustic neuroma) or some other correctable problem. Your physician will also check your circulatory system, thyroid, blood sugar, and blood pressure to determine if they are normal. If any of these are out of whack, getting them under adequate control will allow your vertigo to subside.

However, a fairly common cause of constant vertigo is anxiety. Problems with stress and depression can be manifested by the symptom of dizziness or vertigo. If none of the correctable causes of vertigo is found, your physician should find out if any underlying symptoms of anxiety exist. If you are under undue stress or are experiencing symptoms of depression, the major treatment would be to correct these underlying problems.

LABYRINTHITIS

My doctor tells me I have labyrinthitis. What is this?

Labyrinthitis is an acute inflammation of the inner ear characterized by a rather sudden onset of severe vertigo, usually with marked nausea and vomiting. Any movement, even turning the head, seems to trigger the severe vertigo. The unfortunate part of this problem is that the inflammation or swelling of the inner ear is not cured with antibiotics. The treatment consists of simply having the individual go straight to bed and keep the head from moving as much as possible. (Some people have noted that even turning their head on the pillow can trigger the symptoms.) The doctor will have the person force plenty of fluids and may prescribe a medication to help control the vertigo until it subsides on its own. Acute labyrinthitis will last approximately 4 to 5 days and generally will not cause any permanent damage to the inner ear or hearing mechanism.

NEUROFIBROMATOSIS

What is neurofibromatosis?

Neurofibromatosis (von Recklinghausen's disease) is a disease that causes small to large tumors to develop in the skin, eyes, and central nervous system. These appear as lumps on the skin and can be either benign or malignant.

Neurofibromatosis occurs once in every 3000 births and is transmitted by a dominant gene. It begins with the appearance of 1 or more brownish spots on the body, called cafe-au-lait spots. These are generally followed by the formation of 1 or more tumors under the skin.

There is no cure for von Recklinghausen's disease. Treatment generally consists of excision of the tumors when they become disfiguring and plastic reconstruction. Close monitoring is necessary to see whether any tumors become cancerous. People with von Recklinghausen's disease can suffer anything and everything from a small number of skin tumors to the total disfiguration of the person as portrayed in the movie *The Elephant Man*.

227

SEIZURE

What is epilepsy?

Epilepsy is a disease causing repeated seizures, which are uncontrolled spontaneous discharges from the central nervous system that interfere with normal function. In epilepsy, the brain tissue begins to spontaneously fire off repeated electrical discharges. The symptoms of an epileptic seizure depend upon the extent of the discharge and how much of the brain is involved.

To date, medical science does not know exactly why certain people have epilepsy and others do not. Nor do we know exactly why these brain cells fire off repeatedly. We do know that it is important to distinguish the type of seizures a person is having because that relates directly to the specific treatment to control them.

Seizures are classified as either partial or generalized. Partial seizures are localized in 1 area of the brain and do not involve all the brain tissue. Individuals who suffer from partial seizures will have spontaneous motor activity only in that portion of the body controlled by that particular part of the brain.

Generalized seizures, however, affect larger portions of the brain and cause more widespread symptoms. The most common types of seizures, petit mal and grand mal, are generalized seizures.

Grand mal seizures, also known as major motor seizures, can occur at any age and are characterized by severe tightening and jerking of the whole body. Visually, they last anywhere from 2 to 5 minutes but, in severe cases, can last up to 1 hour. The individual's breathing may stop, and he or she may turn blue. After the seizure is over, the person will resume breathing but will be in a sleepy, almost unconscious state for several minutes to several hours.

Petit mal seizures generally occur between the ages of 4 and 8 and are characterized by episodes of staring during which the child cannot be aroused or of staring spells associated with some jerking or motion. These spells are brief (a few seconds) but may occur as often as 50 to 100 times per day.

Another type of seizure, the psychomotor seizure, is more typical in older children and adults. These seizures vary greatly in how they occur but may involve staring spells combined with lip smacking, confusion, mumbled speech, and bizarre behavior. Again, they usually last only a few minutes but may occur several times a day.

Mild clonic seizures occur principally in infants, most often between 3 and 9 months of age. These seizures are characterized by spasms that result in extreme tightening of the muscles that flex the head. A child may be lying down and have a severe spasm that causes the head to be jerked forward. If the child is sitting, the head will be jerked forward into a drooping position. Individual attacks last only a few seconds, but they frequently occur in clusters, thus appearing to last for several minutes.

A proper diagnosis of the type of seizure must be made before correct treatment can be given.

Are seizures inherited?

According to the Epilepsy Foundation of America, seizures are not inherited in the same way that people inherit the color of their eyes. It is well known, however, that the incidence of seizure disorders tends to run in families. According to *Patient Care* magazine (September 15, 1983), the prevalence of epilepsy in the general population is about 0.5% to 2.0%. In children who have had one parent with epilepsy, this rises to about 6%, while it is 10% to 12% among children whose parents both have had epilepsy. However, many people with a high susceptibility may never develop the condition unless something happens to them during their life that in some way injures their brain. Even though there is a chance that children of a person with epilepsy will eventually develop the condition, it is much more likely that they will not.

If heredity does not cause all seizures, what does?

According to the Epilepsy Foundation of America, in about half of the cases there is no known cause. People who suffer massive head trauma, brain tumors, and strokes have an increased incidence of eventual development of seizure disorders. The more severe the head injury, the greater the chance of developing seizures. According to Dr. Gilbert H. Glason (*Beeson-McDermott Textbook of Medicine*), about 30% to 40% of the people who have had massive head injuries will experience seizures, with a large percentage of those seizures happening within the 1st 2 years after the injury.

After the age of 50, the chance of a tumor being the cause of a seizure is approximately 15%. Hardening of the arteries of the brain is the most common cause of seizures after the age of 50. Also, a small percentage of people who have had strokes ultimately develop seizures. The risk of developing seizures after a stroke is higher if the stroke has been caused by a hemorrhage.

Alcohol withdrawal seizures are another common form of adult seizure. An alcoholic who stops drinking may, within the 1st 7 to 48 hours, develop generalized seizure activity, apparently caused by the effects of alcohol on the brain over a prolonged period of time.

How is epilepsy diagnosed?

The diagnosis of epilepsy depends upon a combination of the history and an appropriate medical evaluation. Getting an exact history of the seizure, including how the individual felt immediately prior to it, is extremely important so that the physician can characterize exactly which type the individual had. Many people will say that they "knew" they were going to have a seizure. Others, because they are unconscious during the seizure, have no recollection before or immediately after its occurrence.

The next most important part of the diagnosis is a thorough medical examination. During this examination, the physician will look for possible causes of seizure disorders, such as hardening of the arteries of the brain, alcoholism, brain tumor, or other changes within the metabolic system of the body. Once these have been ruled out, the physician will want to study brain wave patterns. In order to get a true picture, your physician will order an EEG (electroencephalogram) to trace the electrical discharges of the brain. In many cases, epileptics have characteristic brain wave discharge patterns that can pinpoint the diagnosis, even though they are not currently having a seizure.

Are all seizures really epilepsy?

No. The diagnosis of epilepsy is based on clinical findings, specifically the demonstration of recurrent, stereotypical attacks of altered behavior or general seizure activity. However, epilepsy is not the only condition that can abruptly interrupt normal brain function to produce attacks of disturbed behavior.

The loss of consciousness caused by a decrease in the blood supply to the brain, referred to as syncope, may be confused with epileptic seizures. A simple fainting spell (vasovagal syncope) is heralded by a light-headed feeling, visual grey-out, and ringing in the ears, followed by loss of muscle tone and loss of consciousness.

Breath-holding episodes in infants and children may also be erroneously diagnosed as epilepsy, especially "white" breath-holding attacks in which the child does not turn blue. Although such attacks typically occur in infants, they have been reported in adults.

Abrupt disturbances in behavior are among the most distinctive clinical features of partial seizures. But this type of behavior may be evident in people who suffer from narcolepsy, a severe disorder of normal sleep patterns characterized by irresistible attacks of daytime sleep, hallucinations, and sleep paralysis. Narcolepsy may appear in childhood but more typically begins in adolescence.

People who faint while they are sitting up and do not immediately fall to the ground may also have spontaneous seizure activity. A typical example is a person who faints in a chair and, because the blood supply to the brain is reduced, suffers a generalized seizure but does not have any underlying problems of epilepsy.

PARKINSON'S DISEASE

What is Parkinson's disease?

Parkinson's disease, a condition also known as shaking palsy, was 1st described by James Parkinson in 1817. Since then, we have begun to understand that a deficiency of dopamine and other chemicals within the brain cells causes a complex of symptoms know as parkinsonism.

Parkinson's disease occurs throughout the world in all racial and ethnic groups. Rarely seen in people under 40 years of age, its average onset is around age 60. Approximately 1% of the population over 60 years of age suffers from this disease. Genetic factors have long been suspected of playing a major role, but the evidence doesn't show that parkinsonism is transmitted directly through families. In fact, family studies show that only 2% of the children of Parkinson's disease patients develop it.

The initial symptoms of Parkinson's disease are a very slight weakness and a tendency to tremble, expecially in 1 hand or, less often, in 1 foot. Often the individual will experience slowness or awkwardness in using that particular part of the body. If the arm is affected the person will tend to hold it in a flexed position. Sufferers will also lose some amount of facial expression and have a deliberate quality of speech. The 1st symptoms are usually mild and may persist for up to 2 years. Gradually, however, individuals become more and more affected, and symptoms begin to appear on the other side of the body. Posture becomes less erect, and a characteristic stooped, shuffling gait may develop.

As the disease progresses, all movements of the body become very slow, walking becomes extremely difficult, and the tremor and the tightness of the arms become generalized. There can be tremors of the lips, tongue, jaw, and facial muscles as well as the limb muscles.

In the latter stages, approximately 50% of persons with Parkinson's disease are affected by a gradual dementia. Initially, the person is simply forgetful, but gradually this increases until the person loses touch with reality.

Is there any treatment for Parkinson's disease?

The most effective treatment available is a chemical called levodopa (L-dopa), a chemical similar to the dopamine that is deficient in people with this disease. L-dopa may be given alone but is more often given in combination with other medications that protect the body from some of the side effects of L-dopa.

A variety of other drugs have been used to try to reduce some of the symptoms. These include medications that directly suppress the tremor and also deal with the depression often complicating parkinsonism.

I have a constant tremor. Do I have Parkinson's disease?

Of course, parkinsonism must be considered in anyone with a tremor, especially in a person over 60 years of age. However, a more frequent cause of tremors in younger patients is essential tremor, an inheritable disease characterized by a tremor that can affect the hands, the head, or even the voice. Essential tremors appear to be genetically transmitted. They do not, however, appear to shorten the person's life span and do not have the gradual dementia of parkinsonism. Since there is no known cause for these tremors, attention turns to the possible management.

Individuals with essential tremor are often aware that an alcoholic beverage can temporarily cause the tremor to stop. But even though alcohol stops the tremor for a few minutes or hours, the tremors can recur and be more severe several hours after drinking stops. So, best treatment of benign essential tremors depends on various sedatives and certain tranquilizers. Although the tremor never completely goes away, it can be significantly reduced by these drugs. A newer medication, propranolol, may be more effective in some people, but it has side effects and should be used cautiously.

FAINTING

What causes someone to faint?

Fainting, or syncope, refers to a loss of consciousness associated with a complete loss of muscle tone throughout the body. Although fainting is a common symptom encountered by physicians, patients often confuse fainting with other symptoms. Some patients may think they have fainted when in reality they have been severely dizzy or have had a light-headed, unsteady, or other ill-defined feeling of weakness without true loss of consciousness.

True fainting spells are usually preceded by certain symptoms. Most people will say that they have a feeling of light-headedness accom-

232

panied by sweating, paleness, nausea, and perhaps an inability to think clearly. The person may also be aware of a fluttering of the heart. All of these symptoms occur just prior to losing consciousness.

The causes of fainting can be divided into 2 broad categories. The 1st, vasovagal syncope, occurs in otherwise healthy individuals—as when muscular athletes faint in my office because they had blood drawn. This type of fainting spell occurs due to a sudden increase in stimulation of the vagus nerve. Because of this excess stimulation, the person experiences a sudden drop in blood pressure that results in a decreased oxygen supply to the brain. The heart rate cannot increase fast enough to compensate for this drop, and the person faints.

The 2nd category includes those people who faint not from a stimulation of the vagus nerve but from a decreased blood supply to the brain. People who have high blood pressure and take diuretics sometimes say that if they rise too quickly from a sitting position, they feel sweaty, become nauseated, and pass out. When a person with hypertension stands up, the blood vessels clamp down, forcing blood to the brain. For a hypertensive person on certain medications, the clamping down of the arteries cannot occur as rapidly; therefore, the blood pressure falls, the blood supply to the brain decreases, and the person loses consciousness.

Another common reason for fainting is lack of circulation in the brain arteries. People who have hardening of the arteries of the brain will faint when not enough blood gets to the brain through these diseased arteries.

Other causes of fainting spells have nothing to do with the heart or the brain. People with low blood sugar (hypoglycemia) can also have fainting spells. This generally occurs because of a sudden drop in a person's blood sugar after eating a high-calorie meal. Within 1 to 2 hours, the individual may experience sweating, tremor, confusion, a sudden urge to eat, and occasionally loss of consciousness.

Hyperventilation is another cause of fainting. Usually because of an excessive amount of anxiety, the person will begin to breathe very rapidly. This rapid rate of breathing does not allow enough oxygen to be transferred into the system. The lack of oxygen, in turn, causes a tightening of the arteries of the brain, a decreased blood flow to the brain and fainting.

The treatment of syncopal spells depends upon the exact cause. Anyone who faints, especially if over 60 years of age, should see a physician.

Can you have a fainting spell because of your heart?

In the previous discussion, I mentioned some of the more common causes of fainting spells. However, for individuals with severe heart disease, there can be more complicated problems. People with hardening of the arteries of the heart can sometimes have episodes when the heart rate slows tremendously. This is referred to as bradycardia. When this happens, the normal heart rate, about 70 beats per minute, drops dramatically to 30 or 40 beats per minute, causing a lack of blood and oxygen to the brain. Hence, these people will have weak and fainty spells, usually occurring when they stand up or get out of a chair.

We also know that some people have irregular heart rhythms, or arrhythmias. During an arrhythmic attack, the heart can beat too fast, and just as with too low a heart rate, not enough blood is being pumped with each heartbeat to the brain; thus fainting can result.

DEMENTIA

As my grandmother gets older, she seems to be more confused. What causes this?

This confusion, clinically referred to as dementia, means that there has been impairment of a person's ability to think clearly, be in touch with reality, or carry out normal daily activities. It is caused to some degree by diffuse damage to the brain tissue. Dementia is severe enough in about 5% of the population over 65 years of age to render them unable to cope with the activities of daily living.

There are 2 primary causes of dementia in elderly people: hardening of the arteries of the brain, and Alzheimer's disease. Alzheimer's disease is characterized by the development of plaques (scar tissue) in important parts of the brain cells. Exactly what causes these plaques is currently under debate, but some believe they could be caused by a virus or an antigen-antibody reaction.

The early manifestations of Alzheimer's disease can be extremely subtle and are often more obvious to the families of the patient than to the patient. These people will generally have some change in their personality patterns or may simply be a little forgetful. This forgetfulness can be as subtle as an inability to remember telephone numbers or as obvious as forgetting names of people important to them. At this point in the disease's progress, individuals are generally totally unaware of their inability to remember. They may consider it an inconvenience, but most pay no attention.

As the disease progresses, abnormalities of behavior become more obvious. Relatives find that the individuals are totally unreliable in handling money, conveying messages, and making simple decisions.

They seem to be more accident prone during this stage because they simply forget how to perform routine activities. They may also experience a sense of disorientation and are easily lost when they get away from home.

A more advanced state of Alzheimer's disease renders the person totally unable to perform activities of daily living. The individual has to be dressed, bathed, and fed. Some will lose control of the bladder and rectal sphincters and become incontinent. Others may spend the whole day sitting in a chair and staring at the walls.

During the final stages of Alzheimer's disease, medical complications such as malnutrition, infections and injuries occur that generally lead to death.

This disease affects hundreds of thousands of individuals in our country; there is no cure. However, with the help of Alzheimer's support groups in the local community and through conversations with and literature from the physician, the families of patients with Alzheimer's can better understand the disease, how it affects the patient, and how they can cope with it.

The 2nd most frequent cause of dementia is atherosclerosis of the arteries of the brain. When these arteries get hardened with plaque formations, the flow of blood through these arteries is reduced. This reduced blood supply causes some of the brain tissue supplied by these arteries to malfunction and even die (a stroke). The greater the reduction in blood flow, the greater the damage to the brain tissue.

As this slow yet progressive damage occurs, generally in older patients, the person's ability to concentrate and remember is lost. The common term for this process is *senility*.

How do you evaluate a patient with Alzheimer's disease?

Generally, during the 1st stage of Alzheimer's disease, neither the patient nor the family is concerned enough to seek medical attention. However, as the disease progresses, the family will request that the physician evaluate the patient. Because there is no known cure for Alzheimer's, the evaluation will seek to rule out every other potential cause of dementia. The physician will make sure that the patient does not have any signs of hardening of the arteries, hypertension, thyroid disease, diabetes, or some other potentially correctable problem. At this stage, the physician should make sure that the overall health of the patient is good.

After a thorough physical examination, including a complete neurological evaluation, the patient will probably have a brain or CAT (computerized axial tomography) scan to see if there have been any previous "silent strokes." These silent strokes might have occurred without any other signs or symptoms, but they might have done permanent damage to portions of the brain. When the physical examination is complete, psychological testing can be performed to identify early signs of Alzheimer's. Once the physician is reasonably sure that the patient has Alzheimer's, a counseling session should be held with the family to make sure they understand what effects the disease has and what they can expect in the future.

17.

Headaches

THE "COMMON" HEADACHE

How common are headaches?

Headaches are some of the most common medical problems that have occurred throughout the ages, according to the American Association for the Study of Headache. As early as 5000 years ago, the Chinese were using acupuncture to stop headache pain. In A.D. 200, Galen wrote that a cause of headache was prolonged stimulation of the vagus nerve, which runs from the head to the stomach. Galen theorized that when the body became bloated, the irritation from the stomach was transferred to the head and created pain. In the early stages of European history, headaches were treated by everything from bloodletting to cathartics. So, the problem of the "common" headache has been with us throughout time. Only recently have any major advances been made in determining the cause of and the best treatment for headaches.

It is estimated that 80% of the United States population is affected by headaches at some time, and each year about 42 million headaches are reported to physicians. The cause of these headaches differs from individual to individual, but we do know that there are some specifics the physician must look for in a patient who complains of headache.

Headaches can be caused by diseases of the bones of the skull, an inflammation or irritation of the nerves within the skull, irritation of the lining of the brain, problems with the vascular system of the brain, brain tumors, trauma to the head, or referred pain (pain originating from one part of the body yet felt somewhere else) from the eye, middle ear, sinuses, or neck. However, in many cases, they are caused not by a physical problem but by anxiety or depression.

237

MIGRAINE HEADACHE

What causes migraine headaches?

Migraine headaches are vascular headaches, which means that the primary cause relates to the blood vessels contained within the brain. A migraine commonly occurs on only 1 side of the head, is often associated with a loss of appetite, and most often is accompanied by nausea and vomiting. Many people will say that they can sense when this type of headache is about to occur because they experience strange sensory, mood, or motor disturbances. There is often a tendency within families to have migraine headaches.

The intense pain of a migraine is caused by a very rapid expansion or dilation of the arteries within the brain. These arteries will suddenly expand, then tighten up or constrict, thus creating the typical pain.

It is interesting that many people will say they have migraines even though their headache pattern does not match that of a typical migraine. It was quite common many years ago to be told that any headache was a "migraine," but today physicians realize that most of these headaches are related to tension and are not true vascular headaches. It is very important to make this distinction, because the treatment of a true migraine is entirely different from that of a tension headache.

Are all migraine headaches alike?

For a majority who suffer from migraine headaches, the pattern of the pain will match that of the "classic" migraine. A number of people, however, will suffer a vascular headache without some of the associated classical symptoms. These "common" migraines generally do not have the early warning signs (prodromata) and are less likely to be on just 1 side of the head. These headaches may also be referred to as sick headaches, or atypical migraines, and are most often caused by seasonal, environmental, occupational, menstrual, or other lifestyle changes. Common or atypical migraines can be just as intense as the classic migraine but are more difficult for the physician to diagnose.

How are migraine headaches treated?

Because migraine headaches occur with different intensity and frequency, the treatment will depend upon each individual's specific problems. With the advent of new drugs, physicians are now able to provide treatment that can, in many instances, prevent or at least reduce the severity of recurrent attacks.

238

Once it has begun, a migraine is almost impossible to treat with anything other than pain medications, such as different analgesic combinations, with a mild sedative and/or antinausea medicine.

The classic medication used to prevent migraine is ergotamine. This seems to prevent acute dilation of arteries within the brain and works best when taken immediately upon realizing a migraine attack is about to occur. Ergotamine comes in pill form (to be placed under the tongue) or in tablet form. These tablets can be taken every ½ hour until the headache stops or until the maximum amount, usually six tablets, has been taken within a specific period of time.

Some of the newer medications that can be used on a long-term basis to prevent migraine headaches are the beta-blockers. Instead of having to wait for the onset of a headache, an individual can take these over a long period of time, and they seem to prevent rapid dilation of arteries within the skull. There have also been some advances in the use of medications called calcium antagonists, reported to relieve attacks of migraine in a significant number of people.

The exact prescription and its dosage will depend upon your age, your sensitivity to medication, and the intensity of your attacks. If your symptoms match those of either classic or atypical migraines, you should consult your physician for the proper diagnosis and treatment to help relieve the suffering from these very painful headaches.

What can cause a migraine to occur?

Migraine headaches can be brought on by any number of stimuli, such as staring at a very bright light, having a sinus infection, or having an acute allergic reaction to food, especially protein. Consuming excessive amounts of animal fat or alcohol or missing a meal may also precipitate an attack.

Psychological factors probably play a major role in the frequency of attacks; mental fatigue, anxiety, and stress have all been known to bring on severe headaches.

Hereditary predisposition is also an important factor in migraines, the tendency to suffer from them is inherited directly within families. Migraine headaches can occur at puberty, but most do not manifest themselves until later, in middle life. Children who suffer from severe car sickness and bouts of vomiting for unknown reasons may develop migraines later in life. And, on the whole, women are 7 times more likely to develop migraines than men.

I have heard that you can have a migraine headache that affects only your eyes. Is that true?

An ophthalmic migraine is an unusual form of vascular headache and occurs because the dilation affects only the artery that supplies the eye.

Visual disturbances can occur with an ophthalmic migraine that may last days or even weeks. A paralysis of the 3rd cranial nerve that goes to the eye muscles can cause a temporary paralysis of the muscle, a drooping of the eyelid, or changes in the pupil reaction. If you have these symptoms on the same side as the headache occurs, your physician will want to make sure that they are not caused by more serious problems in your vascular system. If you do not, you probably are having an ophthalmic migraine.

The typical sufferer of an ophthalmic migraine will have an excruciating pain over 1 eye, associated with visual disturbances within the eye. The treatment of an ophthalmic migraine is the same as that of a classic migraine.

TENSION HEADACHE

What causes a tension headache?

Tension headaches (cephalalgia) probably represent over 75% of all headache complaints. They generally occur in response to a constant or periodic emotional upset. Often the person may not even recognize that stress is present.

The pain of tension headaches is caused by a severe tightening of the muscles of the neck and scalp and is often felt in the front of the head, the back of the head, or in the temples. The pain is generally described as steady and constant, and it feels as if the head is caught in a vise. These headaches will generally be located in 1 part of the head and may continue there for weeks, months, or even years.

Tension headaches are almost always related to a specific stress situation. A basic challenge in evaluating people with tension headaches is trying to uncover the underlying stress.

What is the best way to treat a tension headache?

In a tension headache, the most beneficial form of therapy deals with handling the stress or anxiety that caused the headache to occur. Preventive measures include the learning of relaxation and stress-reduction techniques. Many who suffer from tension headaches on a chronic basis have found relief in regular exercise programs that seem to relieve the underlying stress and, therefore, the frequency and intensity of the headaches. The treatment of the actual pain is best accomplished by the use of an analgesic medication, which may contain a mild sedative.

SINUS HEADACHE

How can a sinus problem cause a headache?

Your sinuses are air cavities located within the bones of the skull. As long as they contain only air, no pressure is exerted on the linings of the sinuses, but when pressure builds up from fluid and/or infection, a great deal of pressure can be exerted, and a headache can follow.

Sinus headaches usually start in the front of the head and can also extend under the eyes. Generally, the headache begins early in the morning and subsides in the afternoon or early evening. The intensity is frequently increased by movement of the head, especially when bending down. Anything that increases pressure in the sinuses, such as straining, coughing, or even a tight shirt, can aggravate the headache.

Remember that the sinus headache is a symptom, not a disease. It will only subside when the underlying sinus pressure or infection has been treated, usually through the use of decongestants and antibiotics.

CLUSTER HEADACHE

I've often heard that some headaches occur in clusters. What does that mean?

Headaches that appear in clusters are probably the most excruciating and painful of all the vascular headaches. Referred to as cluster headaches, Horton's syndrome, and histamine cephalalgia, they are terribly severe and occur in frequent attacks of very short duration. People suffering from cluster headaches may have up to 20 severe, short headaches a week that occur at approximately the same time of day. The headaches may then go away and not return for several months or years.

Cluster headaches are generally 1-sided and are associated with a reddening of the white portion of the eye, increased tearing in the eye, a narrowing of the pupil, and increased sweating on that side of the head. These symptoms are caused by a dysfunction in the nerves that control these activities.

There is no tendency for cluster headaches to occur in families. We are not sure why people suffer from them, but their severity has created a great deal of interest in why they occur and how to treat them. We do know, for instance, that attacks of cluster headaches can be precipitated by alcohol, nitrates, or histamines.

Cluster headaches are treated basically the same way as migraine headaches. The chemical ergotamine has been effective for some peo-

241

ple, and a new medication, methysergide, has been used with great success in others.

When should I call my doctor about a headache?

As I have said, approximately 80% of the American population will suffer a headache at some time. The most common cause will be sinus congestion or tension. If you have a headache that responds to fairly normal doses of a mild analgesic such as acetaminophen or aspirin, the chances are that you do not have a severe type of headache. If your headache fails to respond to these types of medication, or if it occurs frequently and interferes with your normal lifestyle, you should consult your physician.

Any time a headache is associated with double vision, severe nausea and vomiting, or a fainting spell, you should contact your physician immediately.

18.

Special Health Problems of Women

CYSTITIS

What is cystitis?

Cystitis, or infection of the bladder, is a common problem for many women; up to 25% of all women will have a bladder infection sometime during their lives.

Cystitis is caused by bacteria normally present in the digestive tract. Even with the best hygiene, these bacteria can sometimes reach the vaginal area. Because there is only a 1″ barrier between the vagina and the urethra, the entrance to the bladder, there's little resistance to the entry of bacteria into the bladder. Once the bacteria enter the bladder, they multiply rapidly, infecting the normally bacteria-free urine.

How can I tell if I have cystitis?

When the bacteria have begun to multiply within the bladder, certain symptoms result. Not all of these will occur, but women with cystitis will notice some of the following:
- A constant desire to urinate, even minutes or seconds after emptying the bladder
- A straining feeling at the end of urination
- Considerable pain or burning during urination
- Burning that increases after having finished urinating
- A feeling that the bladder is not entirely emptied
- A constant desire to urinate and/or having to get up several times during the night to urinate
- A feeling that the flow and the force of the urine are much reduced

If any of these symptoms occur, especially if associated with fever, you should consult your physician.

Are women more susceptible to cystitis than men?

Women usually have more cases of cystitis than men because, as explained earlier, their anatomy offers little resistance to the entrance of bacteria into the bladder. In men, the penis forms a natural barrier between the normal bacteria in the digestive tract and the bladder.

Another reason that women tend to have more bladder infections than men is that during intercourse, the penetration of the man's penis can irritate the woman's bladder stem (urethra), especially in the male-superior position. If a woman does not empty her bladder fairly soon after intercourse, this irritation can cause swelling and eventual infection in the bladder. This, by the way, is *the* cause for the condition known as "honeymoon cystitis."

How is cystitis treated?

Almost all cases of cystitis are caused by a type of bacteria, the most common being *E. coli*. Since 80% to 85% of all bladder infections are caused by this specific bacteria, a physician will prescribe an antibiotic to kill the bacteria at the onset of the symptoms. The antibiotic most frequently used is a sulfa preparation or, if you are allergic to sulfa, a medication such as ampicillin or cephalothin.

These medications may also be combined with a drug called Pyridium, an anesthetic that coats the lining of the bladder and relieves some of the pain and burning. If you take Pyridium alone or in combination with an antibiotic, be warned that it will cause your urine to turn orange. Don't panic—this is a normal reaction. While taking Pyridium, you may want to protect your undergarments and clothes with a minipad, since the dye can permanently stain fabrics.

Should I do anything besides take antibiotics for cystitis?

There's an excellent way to guard against potential infections and to get rid of infections when they occur—drink plenty of liquids. When you drink plenty of liquids, your bladder gets washed out more often because you produce more urine. And the more urine that is formed, the faster the bacteria are excreted.

Don't hold back when you feel you need to urinate. Most women tend to urinate less frequently than they really should, waiting until they finish whatever they are doing, even though they have the urge to empty the bladder. This practice tends to increase the chance of infection, because delaying urination can give the bacteria within the bladder a chance to continue to multiply.

It is also recommended that immediately after sexual intercourse, women empty the bladder so that any irritation that has occurred will not have a chance to set up an infection.

What if I constantly have bladder infections?

A common cause of constant bladder infections is the inability to adequately drain the bladder when urinating. This may be caused by a swelling or an abnormally small opening to the bladder (urethra). If you have confirmed multiple bouts of cystitis, your doctor will generally recommend an evaluation by a urinary tract specialist, a urologist, to find out if your urethra is too small. A simple procedure called a urethral dilatation may need to be done, so that the bladder opening is large enough to empty the bladder during urination.

It is also a possibility that women with frequent infections will need to take antibiotics on a long-term basis. This will completely kill all of the bacteria in the urine and keep the bladder infection free.

Why do some women retain a lot of fluid?

Normally, excess body fluid is carried through the blood system into the kidneys and discarded through urination. But for some women, this fluid seeps out of the bloodstream, collects in the tissues, and causes swelling. This swelling may be around the ankles, causing significant problems with wearing certain shoes. It can be in the hands, making it difficult to take rings off. Or the fluid can be retained in the abdomen, causing a bloated sensation.

No matter how you experience fluid retention, it should be evaluated by your physician. Although many women retain fluids because of the change in hormonal levels, there are other, more serious problems that can cause fluid retention. Your physician will want to make sure that you are not retaining fluid because of abnormalities in your kidney function, heart function, or blood vessels. Once these are proven to be okay, your physician will turn to the symptom itself.

All women who suffer from fluid retention should restrict their daily intake of salt. Salt consumed through the diet eventually gets into the blood system. The more salt in the blood, the more fluid retained to wash it out, so reduction in salt intake will make a significant difference in the amount of fluids retained.

PELVIC INFLAMMATORY DISEASE

What is pelvic inflammatory disease?

According to the Centers for Disease Control, pelvic inflammatory disease (PID) affects an estimated 850,000 women every year. It infects the fallopian tubes, the ovaries, or the uterus itself. But most often the fallopian tubes are involved, and the infection is referred to as acute salpingitis. The symptoms are intense pain in the pelvic area, fever, chills, and sometimes a vaginal discharge.

Pelvic inflammatory disease accounts for approximately 200,000 hospital admissions annually. It requires specific antibiotic treatment and may require surgical intervention.

PID is classified according to the type of organism or bacterium that causes it. Often it is a sexually transmitted organism, such as the organisms causing gonorrhea and chlamydia, but a certain percentage of cases are caused by other bacteria.

PID may develop in any sexually active woman, but it appears to be more frequent in women who have had previous bouts with PID, are less than 20 years old, have multiple sex partners, and have not been pregnant. Some contraceptive techniques, especially intrauterine devices (IUD's), appear to increase the incidence of PID. The use of oral contraceptives, on the other hand, has been shown to significantly reduce the likelihood of PID.

VARICOSE VEINS

What are varicose veins?

Approximately 1 out of every 4 women (and 1 out of every 10 men) suffers from varicose veins. Varicose veins are veins in the leg that become twisted and enlarged because blood collects in them instead of traveling back to the heart. Gravity is the main factor that contributes to their development.

Generally, blood that has circulated to the feet returns to the heart through a special system of valves in the veins. When these valves are damaged, blood can pool in the veins, enlarge them and cause varicose veins.

People with a family history of varicose veins are more prone to develop them.

Can I prevent varicose veins?

In some people, varicose veins will develop no matter what you do, especially if the tendency runs in your family. There are, however, some things you can do to help prevent them, such as the following:

246

- Wear good support stockings when you have to stand for long periods.
- Rest and elevate your legs when possible.
- Avoid being overweight, and reduce your salt intake.
- Exercise regularly. A brief 20- to 30-minute walk or bike ride will strengthen the muscles in your legs and help them return the blood to your heart.

If I have developed them, are there any treatments for varicose veins?

If your varicose veins are in the very early stages, there are some things you can do to help. When you lie down, elevate your legs above the level of your heart so that the veins have a chance to drain. Begin a good exercise program to strengthen your calf muscles. Support your veins and prevent further expansion with proper compression—support hose are best.

If the varicose veins do not respond to these simple measures, there are 2 basic forms of medical treatment: (1) in a surgical procedure that will actually "strip" the veins, some of the more damaged veins can be tied off and removed; and (2) in select cases, the veins may be injected with a chemical cautery that will destroy them without harming the patient.

BREAST LUMPS AND BREAST CANCER

My doctor says that I have fibrocystic breast disease. What does that mean?

Fibrocystic breast disease is the most common benign (noncancerous) breast condition in women of childbearing age; it is characterized by lumps in the breasts that occasionally become very tender, painful, and swollen. This tends to worsen just before the menstrual cycle begins and subsides after the period is over. It is estimated that 1 out of every 5 women between the ages of 25 and 50 will develop this condition.

What causes fibrocystic breast disease?

The cysts appear to be in response to the fluctuating levels of the hormones estrogen and progesterone that regulate the menstrual cycle.

A woman's breast is made up of mammary glands that produce milk in the breast-feeding mother, mammary ducts, in which the milk collects, fatty tissue, and fibrous, thicker tissue. In fibrocystic breast disease, 1 or more cysts form in 1 or both breasts, and the amount of fibrous tissue increases. Sometimes these lumps contain only the fibrous tissue, but many will fill up with fluid, especially during menstruation. These cystic lumps also can change in size and shape during different stages of the menstrual cycle.

The lumps in my breasts get larger during my period and are very painful. What can I do to relieve the pain?

If a cyst in your breast fills up with fluid during your period, the best thing to do is to apply local heat with a hot washcloth or a heating pad for 30 minutes, 3 or 4 times a day. Mild doses of aspirin will also help reduce the pain. As long as the cyst reduces in size and the tenderness goes away immediately following your menstrual period, you probably won't need any further treatment.

However, if the pain continues and a cyst does not resolve after your period, consult your physician. It may be advisable for your physician to perform a procedure called aspiration; after an injection of a local anesthetic, a small needle is inserted into the breast directly into the cyst. In this way, the fluid is withdrawn, the cyst is reduced, and the pain should subside.

Do these breast cysts turn into cancer?

In most cases, no. Many studies have tried to determine if there is any correlation between severe fibrocystic disease and the development of cancer. A study of 7000 women in Great Britain failed to show any significant relationship between the occurrence of fibrocystic disease and the risk of cancer, and other studies have subsequently confirmed this finding. However, the condition of women who have severe fibrocystic disease and also have significant risk factors for the development of breast cancer should be watched closely by a physician. Breast self-examination is complicated by the presence of multiple nodules or cysts within the breasts, and any small, cancerous lumps would be difficult for the woman herself to identify.

If I have a lump in my breast, how can my doctor be sure that it isn't cancer?

In many instances, a doctor can tell by simply examining the cyst. If the lesion is suspicious, a doctor can aspirate the cyst, and the fluid that is removed from it is then examined under a microscope. In most cases, it will not be cancerous.

If no fluid is aspirated but there is some doubt about the nature of a lump, your physician may perform a mammogram or may refer you to a surgeon for a biopsy. A biopsy is a procedure where, under sterile conditions, the cyst or a portion of it is removed and thoroughly analyzed under a microscope by a cell specialist or pathologist. In this way, a definite diagnosis can be made as to whether it is cancerous or benign.

If I have a lot of cysts, can I do anything to reduce the problem?

Many women find that if they eliminate certain substances from their diet, they are less apt to have pain and tenderness or develop more cysts. The specific substances that seem to have an effect on cyst formation are those containing caffeine and a similar chemical called methylxanthine.

Coffee, tea, and most cola drinks have a great deal of caffeine in them. Many nonprescription and prescription drugs contain methylxanthine. For instance, a drug commonly used for asthma, theophylline, is high in methylxanthine. Chocolate should also be avoided, since it contains a form of methylxanthine. Here is a list of beverages, foods, and drugs you should avoid if you have fibrocystic disease:

Foods	Prescription Drugs	Nonprescription Drugs
Chocolate	Cafergot	Anacin
Cocoa	Darvon	Bromo Seltzer
Coffee	Empirin with codeine	Dristan
Colas	Fiorinal	Midol
Tea	Percodan	No-Doz
	Soma	Stanback
	Synalgos	Vanquish
	Theophylline	

Taking high doses of vitamin E to alleviate the discomfort of fibrocystic disease has been recommended, since some studies show that large doses of this vitamin can bring significant relief and may even curtail the disease process itself. Because this is somewhat controversial, you should seek advice from your physician regarding his or her view on its potential benefits.

Another recent study shows that cigarette smoking can increase a woman's chance of having painful cysts in her breasts because it stimulates breast tissue growth. Therefore, smoking should also be stopped.

How important is it that I perform breast self-examination?

Breast self-examination is essential for every woman because it is the most frequent way lumps that could signal the presence of breast cancer are found. Women should examine their breasts once a month, at the same time each month. The best time is somewhere between 5 and 7 days after your menstrual flow has stopped. Your physician or local cancer society will be glad to teach you the technique of breast self-examination. You may feel frustrated or even alarmed when you begin to do a breast self-examination because your breasts will feel lumpy all over. But with experience, you will be able to distinguish between the usual lumpiness and a lump that has formed between examinations.

What you are doing is noting any changes from month to month. If you do find a lump, you are *not* to take the responsibility of deciding whether or not you have breast cancer. Contact your physician immediately so that he or she can examine your breasts and determine what should be done.

Can I have my breasts operated on to remove these cysts?

It is rarely done, but surgery called subcutaneous mastectomy can be performed. During this procedure, the surgeon removes most of the breast tissue lying under the skin and replaces it with silicone implants. Women who suffer severe pain from fibrocystic disease, have a strong family history of breast cancer, or have breast cysts diagnosed as likely to develop into cancer may choose to have this procedure performed. This surgery is not for every woman with breast cysts and certainly should not be used to avoid the "nuisance" of examining your breasts.

How common is breast cancer?

Breast cancer is the most common malignancy in women, accounting for 27% of all cancers. Approximately 1 out of 11 American women will develop breast cancer during her life.

We know that certain women are much more prone to develop breast cancer than others and that some factors seem to increase the risk of developing it. Of course, just because a factor is present does not mean that you will have breast cancer; it just means you are in a higher-risk category.

- Having your 1st child after age 35 or never getting pregnant increases your risk 3 to 4 times.
- Over 80% of breast cancers occur in women over 50 years old, which seems to indicate that your age and your having gone through menopause put you at risk.
- The longer you've been having your period, the greater the odds of your developing breast cancer.
- If a family member, especially your mother, developed breast cancer at an early age, you could be a candidate, too.

- Being obese or having diabetes or hypertension seems to be a risk factor.
- A previous history of cancer in 1 breast means that the other breast could be affected.
- Having had cancer of an ovary, the colon, or the lining of the uterus (endometrium) places you at risk for breast cancer.

It is somewhat reassuring to know that more than 70% of all masses, nodules, or lesions found in the breasts are *not* malignant. They are caused by fibrocystic disease, fibroadenomas (benign tumors of connective tissues), papillomas (skin, epithelial, or glandular benign tumors), and sometimes, just fatty tissue.

MAMMOGRAM

What is a mammogram?

Mammography is a means of detecting and evaluating breast lumps with an x-ray that takes pictures (mammograms) of the distinguishing characteristics of noncancerous (benign) and malignant lumps.

Mammography is simple, relatively painless, and carries little or no risk. However, the breast must be compressed firmly while taking the x-ray, and you will probably want to schedule your test when you know your breasts are less tender.

Many women are reluctant to get a mammogram because they feel the radiation exposure significantly increases their chances of developing breast cancer. Mammography, however, has improved greatly over the last several years, and the amount of radiation required to get an adequate picture has been significantly reduced. Only 1 rad is transferred during the taking of a mammogram, and recent studies show that this does not increase the risk of developing breast cancer. (RAD refers to "radiation absorbed dose" and is equal to sunlight exposure of standing outdoors for 1 hour a day for about 2 years. This small amount of absorbed radiation is far outweighed by the diagnostic benefits of mammography.) Most physicians feel that the radiation received from the test is insignificant compared to the benefits of early cancer detection.

If I have no risk factors for developing breast cancer, how often should I get a mammogram?

Mammography is not recommended for nonrisk women under the age of 35. Between the ages of 35 and 40, every woman should get 1 baseline mammogram and between the ages of 40 and 50, women should get mammograms every 2 to 3 years, depending upon individual health problems. After age 50, it is recommended that women have a yearly mammogram for the detection of early, more curable, breast cancer.

Communicating closely with your physician is essential to set up a schedule for breast self-examination, physician examination, and periodic mammogram if you are at risk for developing breast cancer.

Does a mammogram tell me whether or not I have cancer?

Yes and no. Some characteristic findings during mammography can signal high probability of the presence of a cancer. There are also more subtle findings that make a physician suspect that a particular nodule is cancerous. What you need to remember is that mammography is *part* of the evaluation for potential breast cancer. In a small percentage of people, the mammogram is definite, but for most people, it is an adjunct to the physician's examination and other tests.

MENOPAUSE

What is menopause?

Menopause marks the end of a woman's reproductive ability. The term is derived from 2 Greek words: *menos* (month) and *pauein* (to cause to cease). The Greeks felt this phenomenon happened all at once, but we now know that menopause is, in most women, a gradual thing.

When a woman is between the ages of 45 and 50, for really unknown reasons, her ovaries stop producing the female hormone estrogen. It seems that from the time of a female's birth, each ovary has a certain maximum potential for producing estrogen. Once this potential is reached, the ovaries simply stop producing it. This lack of estrogen causes the physical and emotional changes of menopause.

A woman's cycle will change at the onset of menopause in 1 of 3 ways. (1) Many women will simply have a regular monthly cycle until a certain age, then stop having periods altogether. This is the less frequent, but perhaps most desirable, occurrence. (2) Other women will notice that sometime between the ages of 45 and 50, their periods become more irregular, perhaps coming closer together with a heavier flow. (3) Some women will notice that instead of a 28- to 30-day cycle, their cycles extend to every 35 to 45 days, then skip 1, 2, or more months, until the periods stop. Menopause has occurred when a woman's periods have stopped for at least 6 months to a year.

What are some of the physical symptoms of menopause?

252

About 90% of the women who go through menopause will experience feelings of being very hot and flushed, night sweats, or almost continuous feelings of hot and cold. These feelings, called hot flashes, are caused by a deficiency of estrogen in the bloodstream. Also, because of the lack of estrogen in the system, many women may notice a dryness in the vagina and may have vaginal itching. Because of this condition, called atrophic vaginitis, women experiencing menopause will often complain of pain on intercourse. Another common physical change that women encounter is insomnia, a dramatic change in sleep patterns. Other less frequent occurrences during menopause are constipation, nonspecific aches and pains, headaches, and frequency of urination.

Why do so many women have emotional changes during menopause?

Many women may go through menopause without any emotional difficulty and may experience a sense of freedom from the possibility of an unwanted pregnancy and from a monthly period. In some cases, though, a woman can experience nervousness, irritability, fatigue, or mild depression. These are not usually serious conditions and can be linked to the hormonal deficiencies that occur during menopause. Remember also that menopause usually occurs at a time in a woman's life when many other external changes are taking place. In some cases, the children in the family may be leaving home and making families of their own. The husband might be spending a great deal of his time climbing the corporate ladder or may have midlife adjustments of his own. Women who have never married may also be going through an emotional adjustment to the fact that their chance of ever bearing children is gone forever.

Menopause sometimes triggers changes in the way a woman feels about herself sexually. Women who are taught that sexuality cannot be separated from the ability to bear children may have difficulty adjusting to this time when they are still sexually alive but not fertile. Others may feel that menopause means they are old and, therefore, unattractive. Of course, there are specific problems, such as dryness in the vagina that can cause pain on intercourse, but women should not feel that sexuality stops with the onset of menopause. If you are experiencing this symptom, ask your physician about additional lubrication in the form of a cream or jelly. If a woman has had enjoyable sexual relations before menopause, the years after menopause should be just as enjoyable.

Understanding many of the emotional symptoms can be aided by a firm understanding of the actual chemical changes that are taking place.

Many husbands simply do not understand what is going on during this period of time and become irritable and unsympathetic with their wives. Good communication between the wife, her physician, and her husband is essential.

ESTROGEN REPLACEMENT THERAPY

How are the symptoms of menopause treated?

Remember that the primary physical change during the menopausal years is the cessation of estrogen production; therefore, some of the major symptoms and body changes can be helped by replacing estrogen. Physicians often prescribe it for women when the symptoms of menopause interfere with their normal lifestyles.

Estrogen replacement therapy seems to be particularly effective in treating hot flashes, vaginal irritation, and osteoporosis (the loss of calcium in the bones).

Estrogen replacement therapy can also relieve some of the emotional problems that can occur. Many women experience a decrease in their irritability, anxiety, and depression with estrogen replacement therapy. Today many physicians will prescribe not just estrogen, but a combination of estrogen and another hormone, progestin. While taking this combination of medications, many women will experience a very light "period" at the end of each cycle.

I'm afraid of the side effects of estrogen, especially cancer.

Many women who take estrogen have absolutely no side effects, but a small percentage do suffer some side effects which may be any or all of the following:
- Fluid retention
- Swelling
- Irritability
- Abdominal cramping
- Breast tenderness

Many women reject estrogen replacement therapy because of the fear of cancer. Maybe it's time to set the record straight on the relationship between estrogen and cancer.

All women should be aware that there is some increased risk of developing cancer of the lining of the uterus (endometrium) with the use of estrogen. The risk of endometrial cancer, however, is significantly reduced by combining a lower dose of estrogen with progestin.

Another misconception is that taking estrogen actually increases the risk of developing breast cancer. Studies now indicate that this is not true. In fact, some evidence suggests that there is a *lower* incidence of many forms of cancer in women who take estrogen.

However, estrogen therapy is not for everyone. If you have a history of breast cancer or cancer involving a reproductive organ, if you have had vaginal bleeding that is not a normal period, or if you have any problems with your blood-clotting mechanism, you should talk to your doctor about other ways to deal with the symptoms of menopause.

If I decide to use estrogen, how will I take it?

There are 2 ways that estrogen, or estrogen combined with progestin, can be given. The 1st is in the form of a long-acting injection given every 4 to 6 weeks. This course of action is not convenient for most women and is generally not elected by most physicians.

The 2nd (and most common) way to take estrogen is in pill form. The physician will elect to keep the woman on the estrogen pill throughout the month or stop the pill 5 to 7 days every month. Estrogen is effective in relieving some of the symptoms of menopause only when it is taken on a *regular* basis. Saving up your estrogen pills until you have a hot flash is neither smart nor effective.

A word of caution to women who take a combination of estrogen and progestin. The estrogen pills are taken daily for the 1st 23 to 25 days of the month; during the last 10 to 13 of these days, a progestin pill is taken along with the estrogen. During the days when no estrogen pills are taken, there may be some bleeding similar to your normal menstrual period. This bleeding is of no consequence, and even though it should be reported to your physician, it is a result of the medications being stopped. This bleeding does *not* mean that you are able to get pregnant.

If I have hot flashes and don't take estrogen, what else can I do?

You can do several things to cope with the discomfort of hot flashes. Here are some suggestions:
- Drink ice water when you feel a flash coming on.
- Try cooling yourself with a fan or stand in front of an air conditioner.
- Splash cold water on your face.
- Take a cold shower.
- Wear cotton instead of nylon or other synthetic fibers.
- Wear layered clothing in the winter so that you can remove clothing when a flash occurs.
- Try to avoid situations that seem to provoke hot flashes. For some women, these include undergoing a lot of stress, doing vigorous exercise, eating spicy foods, eating too fast, or drinking alcoholic beverages.

255

Following these suggestions won't cure your hot flashes, but it can help you adjust to them in case you can't take estrogen therapy.

OSTEOPOROSIS

What is osteoporosis?

Osteoporosis is a disease found in 1 out of 4 American women over the age of 50 that is characterized by a thinning of the bones, making them brittle and more vulnerable to fractures.

Our bones are made up of calcium and phosphorus crystals imbedded in protein. Calcium is responsible for the strength and rigidity of bones. The chemicals that contribute to the ability of calcium to make our bones strong are our sex hormones—estrogen in women and testosterone in men.

After menopause, because of the decline in estrogen levels, women's bones tend to lose their calcium. This, combined with a decrease in the amount of calcium in the diet, causes bones to be more brittle and susceptible to fractures.

Osteoporosis affects approximately 20 million people in the United States and is 9 times more common in women than in men. Some people are more susceptible than others; fair-skinned women and women with ancestors from northern Europe, the British Isles, Japan, or China are genetically predisposed to developing osteoporosis. Osteoporosis also tends to run in families. If an individual's close relatives (especially the mother or grandmother) developed frequent fractures, broke a hip, or began to get smaller in stature with age, that individual is more susceptible to developing osteoporosis.

According to the National Institute of Health, about 1.3 million women over the age of 65 will suffer spontaneous fractures because of their brittle bones, the most serious type being a fracture of the hip. In the United States, 80% of the people who sustain hip fractures (200,000 a year) have osteoporosis. Approximately 20% of women who develop hip fractures after the age of 65 will die from complications related to the fracture.

How can I tell if I am developing osteoporosis?

Until recently, it has been difficult to diagnose osteoporosis early enough to make a difference. For instance, conventional x-rays do not pick up the signs of osteoporosis until the loss of bone density reaches about 35%. That is too late.

Many times people have not found out they had osteoporosis until they began to develop some of the painful, disfiguring, and debilitating side effects of the disease. Some of these cases were women who noticed that they were beginning to get smaller as they got older. Loss of calcium in the bones of the spine can lead to a stooped posture called dowager's hump, with a loss in height of as much as 5″ to 8″.

Recently, there have been some significant technological advances that may diagnose osteoporosis at a very early stage. New x-ray equipment called a photon absorptiometry is reported to be able to detect losses of calcium at approximately 1%.

How can osteoporosis be prevented?

Although osteoporosis is thought of as a disease of women over 65, it has its beginning as early as 30 to 35 years of age. The best way to prevent osteoporosis is to build strong bones before the age of 35, keep those bones strong, and maintain calcium levels.

Most experts feel that osteoporosis can be prevented but cannot be reversed if it is already present. There are 3 ways women can help their bones stay strong and full of calcium as they get older.

1. To reduce the risk of developing osteoporosis, women should, at a very young age, increase the amount of calcium they have in their diets. This can be accomplished by increasing the amount of calcium-rich foods they eat, such as kale, spinach, turnip greens, raw oysters, sardines, and canned salmon. The greatest source of calcium, however, is in dairy products such as milk and cheese. The average daily requirement of calcium in premenopausal women is approximately 1000 mg per day.

After age 45, women should increase the intake of calcium to about 1500 mg per day. Most women find it difficult to take in this much calcium through normal diet, so they may opt to take calcium supplements to increase the amount of calcium deposited in the bones.

The process of getting calcium from food into the bones is helped by taking vitamin D. Vitamin D, therefore, should also become part of the replacement therapy and is, in fact, combined with many of the commercial calcium preparations.

2. Any type of physical exercise helps slow down the rate of bone loss associated with osteoporosis. All women should exercise regularly, especially after age 40.

3. There is no direct link between cigarettes, alcohol, and osteoporosis, but a high percentage of women who have osteoporosis are or have been smokers. Some studies also show that excessive amounts of alcohol may increase the risk of developing osteoporosis. It would seem advantageous, therefore, to stop smoking and to reduce alcohol intake.

257

Once I develop osteoporosis, is there any way to treat the disease?

Treatment of osteoporosis, once it has occurred, is geared toward stopping or slowing the progress of the disease. This may include an increase in calcium supplements, estrogen replacement therapy (if medically safe), physical therapy, and exercise.

Each day women who are 45 and older should drink at least 6 glasses of milk or consume the equivalent in other high-calcium foods. This should be combined with a small supplement of vitamin D. Women who find it difficult to take in this much calcium can take oral calcium supplements. Since estrogen therapy seems to be the most effective way of slowing bone loss in postmenopausal women, many doctors will prescribe estrogens in very low doses for women over the age of 45, occasionally in combination with progestin.

Exercise is essential. If you are bedridden, confined to a wheelchair, or in any way restricted in your normal movements, you should receive physical therapy on a regular basis. Walking is excellent for mobile people who cannot do strenuous exercises.

How much calcium do I need to prevent osteoporosis?

The United States recommended daily allowance (RDA) of calcium for women over 19 is approximately 1000 mg per day. Many experts feel that bone loss is significantly reduced if this is increased to 1200 to 1500 mg a day, especially after menopause.

Can you take too much calcium?

An extremely high level of calcium can increase your risk of kidney stones, but this occurs only if you take over 2000 mg a day. That's extremely hard to do—no matter how much milk you drink. But if you have a history of kidney stones, it's best to consult your physician about the amount of calcium you take.

Don't I get enough calcium in my regular diet?

Most women get only about 500 mg per day of calcium through diet. Perhaps that's why the occurrences of osteoporosis are increasing—women live longer, and their calcium-poor diets are starting to catch up with them. And contrary to what a lot of people think, most vitamins—even the supervitamin pills—don't have enough calcium in them to prevent osteoporosis.

Why types of calcium tablets are available as a supplement?

When you look for calcium supplements in your drugstore or health food store, you'll see that there are many different types of calcium products in many different forms. Your options will include calcium lactate, calcium chloride, calcium gluconate, calcium levulinate, and calcium carbonate. Different products have different advantages and disadvantages. Your best bet is to talk with your physician to make sure you choose the right product and the proper dosage.

I've heard that I can take Tums and get enough calcium.

Tums, an antacid whose primary component is calcium carbonate, can be used as a calcium supplement. The distinct advantage of this is the inexpensive nature of Tums. Two Tums per day will satisfy the minimum 1000 mg calcium requirement.

19.

Women's Health

MENSTRUATION

What causes my menstrual cycles to occur?

Your 1st menstrual period, a signal that your body is growing up, usually begins anywhere from 9 to 13 years of age. Menstruation is part of your body's process that prepares you for pregnancy. The 1st signs that your menstrual cycle is ready to begin are the enlargement of your breasts and the growth of hair in your underarms and pubic area. All of these changes are a normal part of becoming an adult, a process called puberty.

Menstruation is controlled by hormones produced in your brain and in your ovaries. (Hormones are chemicals that regulate certain body functions.) The hormones from your ovaries are produced by follicles contained within the ovaries. Each of these follicles has a small egg, or ovum. Although your ovaries contain thousands of these follicles, only a few of them will develop to maturity each month.

Your menstrual cycle occurs in several stages during the month.

Stage 1. The 1st day of your menstrual flow is Day 1. For the next 4 to 7 days, the endometrium, or lining of your uterus, will shed. During this time, you will have light to heavy bleeding and, perhaps, some cramping. The purpose of this portion of your cycle is to dispose of the old lining of the uterus, preparing you for the possibility of getting pregnant.

Stage 2. About the 5th to 7th day of your period, the bleeding will subside, and your body will begin to increase its production of the hormone estrogen. In response to the estrogen, the lining of the uterus begins to get thicker and full of blood vessels.

Stage 3. Your body will continue to produce estrogen for approximately 14 days. Then, 1 of the follicles in 1 of your ovaries bursts and releases an egg. This is known as ovulation.

Stage 4. The egg drops down and enters the fallopian tube that connects the ovary and the uterus.

Stage 5. As the egg travels down the fallopian tube (for the possibility of being fertilized with sperm), the ruptured follicle begins to secrete another female hormone—progesterone.

Stage 6. Progesterone increases the blood supply to the uterus and improves the chances of pregnancy occurring if sperm are present.

Stage 7. If at this time the egg is not fertilized, it will soon break down. At the same time, the follicle in the ovary stops producing progesterone.

Stage 8. The loss of this progesterone level coupled with a slowly declining estrogen level causes the lining of the uterus to break down and pass out of the body. Menstruation begins, and the whole process starts again.

I have a lot of pain with my periods. Is that normal?

Since your uterus contracts to help shed the old lining, it is not unusual to have discomfort during your period. The degree of discomfort, or pain, will vary with each woman. Many times, it is simply an occasional uncomfortable, crampy feeling in your lower stomach the 1st day or 2 of menstruation. This pain usually responds to acetaminophen and a heating pad or hot-water bottle placed on your lower abdomen; a little exercise often helps, too.

However, some women experience a severe amount of cramping and pain during the 1st day or 2 of their periods. This pain can be severe enough for women to miss work or school and have to go to bed until the cramping stops. When the pain is this intense, you should consult your physician. He or she will make sure there is no underlying problem and will probably prescribe medications to ease the pain.

IRREGULAR PERIODS

I'm 35 years old and occasionally have some irregularity with my periods. Is that cause for alarm?

Throughout the childbearing years, women will have an occasional change in their normal menstrual pattern. This might include skipping a month or having the periods come more frequently. This is entirely normal and occurs in about 75% of all women.

As a woman gets older, especially after age 35 or 40, some significant changes can take place in her normal pattern. Women who have had a cycle every 28 days for years will find that their cycle occurs every 21 to 25 days. Also, women who have been relatively pain-free during their periods for many years may develop an increase in cramping as they get older.

Most of these changes are entirely normal, but any change should be reported to your physician. Never assume that a change in the way your body works is just because you're getting older. Let your physician make sure.

My periods are very heavy, painful, and irregular. Is there anything I can do?

Any woman who has heavy, painful, irregular periods should consult her physician to make sure that there is no underlying problem with the ovaries or uterus. If there's no underlying condition and your Pap smear is normal, then your physician can place you on a treatment for this bothersome condition.

Many women, especially those under 35, benefit from chemical cycling of the periods through the use of birth control pills. With the advent of the lower estrogen pills, cycling could significantly reduce the pain and irregularity of your periods without a lot of side effects. If a woman is over 35 and is having an excessive amount of bleeding (especially irregular bleeding), the physician will want to make sure that the lining of the uterus, or endometrium, is normal. This can be determined through the use of a simple suction device or by a surgical scraping procedure known as a D and C (dilation and curettage). Your physician will recommend treatment based on the findings.

Is it abnormal for a teenager's menstrual cycle to be irregular?

Very few teenagers will begin their periods and then maintain a normal cycle. Most are irregular for 3 to 4 years. This means that you can have a period every 4 to 6 weeks, skip a month, or sometimes bleed every 2 weeks. This is not a cause for alarm, unless this irregularity continues after the age of about 15. If this is the case, you may want to consult your physician to see what might cause the continued irregularity.

My doctor wants to put me on birth control pills to regulate my periods. Is that advisable?

If the irregularity of a woman's periods is so pronounced that it interferes with her normal lifestyle, or if cramping is very severe and does

262

not respond to normal medications, a physician may elect to try the woman on birth control pills. Regulating the periods through the use of birth control pills significantly reduces the cramping pain of menstruation for many women.

I do not believe it's wise to try this approach until after the 14th or 15th birthday and only then if the pain and the irregularity are so severe that the young woman cannot function for several days.

What are some of the newer drugs that are used for the control of menstrual pain?

About 30% to 50% of American women of childbearing age suffer from severe pain called dysmenorrhea, the severe cramping during the menstrual period caused by the chemicals (prostaglandins) released by the uterus. It has recently been found that certain medications called prostaglandin inhibitors, which are used in treating arthritis, can help control this pain. Studies show that when properly used, these medications have provided significant relief for 75% of women with this problem. Prostaglandin inhibitor medications are taken approximately 3 to 4 days before the onset of the menstrual period and through the 1st day of the menstrual flow.

If you suffer from severe pain during your period, consult your physician about the possibility of using these new drugs to relieve menstrual pain.

CONTRACEPTIVES

If I need birth control, what options are open to me?

Before a woman chooses to begin sexual activity, she should make the decision to seek birth control advice, if the sexual activity is not intended to result in pregnancy. In the United States today, there are 3 main methods of temporary birth control: oral contraceptives; intrauterine devices (IUD's); and barrier methods (diaphragms, sponges, condoms). We will briefly discuss each method and its current use, reliability, and potential side effects.

1. Oral contraceptives. The year 1985 marked the 25th anniversary of the introduction of oral contraceptives—birth control pills. Even though millions of women have utilized this medication as their choice for birth control, it is still a misunderstood method. A recent Gallup poll found that approximately 75% of the women surveyed believed that there were "substantial" risks associated with the pill, feelings that were founded during the early years when the pill had a much higher

263

estrogen content than now. Today, birth control pills have lower estrogen content and fewer side effects. Some studies show that they actually have many benefits—and the pill is still 99% effective.

2. Intrauterine devices (IUD's). The IUD is the birth control method
chosen by more than 2 million women and is 2nd only to the pill in
effectiveness. The IUD is inserted into the uterus and left in place for a
maximum of 2 years. No one is exactly sure how the IUD works, but it
prevents the implantation of a fertilized egg within the uterus.

IUD's were widely used until the 1970s when the Dalkon Shield, an
all-plastic device, was said to be responsible for severe infections, infertility, and even implicated in some deaths. Since then all Dalkon Shields
have been removed from the market.

Perhaps the most common side effect from the use of IUD's is an
increase in infections. These infections may just cause an increase in
vaginal discharge or may be very severe and cause pelvic inflammatory
disease, which is associated with an increased rate of infertility. An
IUD user frequently has a slightly heavier period and may have increased cramping. In order for the devices to be safe and effective, an
IUD user should get regular checkups from her physician. For the
above reasons, one leading producer, Searle, has recently announced
plans to discontinue production of its IUD. Certainly, IUD's are rapidly
declining as the choice of many women for birth control.

3. Barrier methods. The diaphragm is the primary example of the barrier method of contraception. Approximately 2 million women in the
United States now use a diaphragm—a rubber, dome-shaped device
used with spermicidal jelly and inserted before intercourse. When
properly positioned within the woman's pelvis, the diaphragm completely covers the opening of the womb (cervix). This effectively blocks
penetration by sperm. If any do get past the barrier, the cream or jelly
inserted in and around the diaphragm kills them. Diaphragms must be
fitted by a physician, and they have an effective rate of approximately
75% to 80%.

There are relatively few side effects with the diaphragm, but some
women may be allergic to the rubber coating or to the spermicidal jelly.
Because of the way the diaphragm fits inside the vagina, some women
report an increase in bladder infections. Generally, however, diaphragms are regarded as 1 of the safest methods of contraception as
long as they are not left in more than 24 hours. But to be effective,
diaphragms *must* be left in for at least 6 to 8 hours *after* intercourse.

Recently, a new form of barrier contraceptive, the sponge, has been
introduced. Unlike the diaphragm, the 2″ diameter disposable sponge
fits everyone and does not require fitting by a physican. Made of soft

polyurethane, the sponge contains a widely used spermicide. The sponge is moistened with water to activate the spermicide and inserted to fit against the cervix. The walls of the vagina hold the sponge in place. Once the sponge is inserted, protection from pregnancy begins immediately, and lasts up to 24 hours, when it must be replaced.

The sponge is said to have about an 80% to 85% protection rate from pregnancy. The only side effects are reactions from women who are allergic to the components in the sponge or reactions from their partners, who may also be allergic.

The last form of barrier contraceptive is the condom and an accompanying spermicidal foam. The condom is still the primary birth control method used by over 4 million men.

I've heard that the pill has some very dangerous side effects.

When the birth control pill was introduced, it contained a high amount of the hormone estrogen, and this high-dose estrogen pill was associated with some very serious side effects. Many women experienced fluid retention, elevation of blood pressure, inflammation of the veins (thrombophlebitis), and even the formation of clots that moved to the lung (a pulmonary emboli).

It is unfortunate that many women identify today's birth control pill with yesterday's pill and its side effects because today's low-dose estrogen pills really have fewer side effects.

Perhaps the most bothersome side effect from the low-dose pill is breakthrough bleeding. The estrogen content of the pill is not enough to suppress bleeding during the cycle, and a woman will begin to spot or flow about halfway during her cycle. This side effect, if minimal, can be tolerated or can be improved by changing pills.

The truth is that the new birth control pills probably prevent more complications than they cause, but it is critical that the pill be tailored to the individual. Some women will experience side effects on 1 form of pill but not with another. If you need the protection of a birth control pill, do not hesitate to discuss its effectiveness and potential complications with your doctor.

I have heard that the birth control pill can actually have some positive benefits.

That's true. Not only is it 99% effective in preventing pregnancy, but studies show that a low dosage of estrogen tends to reduce a woman's chances of developing pelvic inflammatory disease, benign breast disease, and ovarian cysts. In fact, the *Journal of the American Medical*

265

Association reported that there seems to be a lower incidence of cancer of the ovaries and uterus in women who take oral contraceptives.

Also, oral contraceptives do not increase the risk of breast cancer. In a controlled study, the use of oral contraceptives did not increase the risk of breast cancer in women considered at high risk—those with fibrocystic disease, those with a family history of breast cancer, or those who had previously used high-estrogen oral contraceptives.

Does using the pill increase my chances of having heart disease?

For women over 35 who also smoke, taking the pill does seem to increase the chances of developing hypertension and high lipid (fats) levels in the blood. Because there is a direct association between cholesterol and hardening of the arteries of the heart, these potential risk factors seem to indicate that the use of birth control pills can increase the risk of heart disease for those women.

However, if a woman stops smoking before taking birth control pills, and if the pills are not taken by women with existing high blood pressure or a family history of heart disease or who are over the age of 35, then the chance of developing heart disease is significantly reduced.

PREMENSTRUAL SYNDROME

What is premenstrual syndrome?

Premenstrual syndrome, or PMS, is a group of symptoms that occur in certain women immediately before their periods and go away after the period begins. According to Guy E. Abraham, M.D., an authority in PMS, this condition will at some time affect approximately 75% of all women during their childbearing years. Approximately 5% to 10% of women suffer symptoms severe enough to interfere with normal existence.

Is PMS real, or is it just a "fad" disorder?

Because of the amount of media attention that has been given to this subject, and because of unethical approaches that have been taken toward its cure, PMS has become somewhat of a fad disease. However, PMS is a legitimate medical concern, and for some women, it is a very serious disease that interferes with family, social, and professional life. For these women, PMS is certainly not a fad disorder; it's a real problem. For many years, unfortunately, women's health problems have been treated differently from those of men. Only recently have a few health professionals recognized the importance of dealing with PMS.

How can I be sure that I have PMS?

Although there is no absolute symptom of PMS, the most common characteristics are depression, fatigue, irritability, anxiety, headaches, breast swelling and tenderness, bloating, weight gain, change in appetite, and craving for sweets. Having 1 or a combination of these symptoms could mean that you are suffering from PMS.

These symptoms will occur anywhere from 2 weeks to 5 days before your period. If they go away almost magically once your period begins, then you probably are suffering from PMS.

It is strongly recommended that any woman who has these symptoms keep a daily record of exactly when during her cycle they occur. If, after several months, you find that they take place only during a specific premenstrual time, and you have a week to 2 weeks with no symptoms after your period, then you probably do have premenstrual syndrome.

What if I have these symptoms all month long?

If you have any or all of these symptoms all month, then you do not have premenstrual syndrome. Check with your physician to see if the symptoms are related to an excessive amount of fluid gain, a problem with your blood sugar, underlying anxiety or depression, or some other hidden condition.

Whether you have PMS or whether your symptoms occur throughout your cycle, if they are persistent, you should consult your physician. It is critical that he or she determine the underlying cause and try to institute a therapy that might provide relief.

What causes PMS?

The exact cause of PMS still remains a mystery. Because PMS varies so widely among women and because there is no absolute set of criteria to make a diagnosis, the research studies in progress often only add to the controversy surrounding the cause or causes of this disorder. There are, however, some theories about the mechanisms that *could* contribute to PMS.

1. Altered endorphin levels. Premenstrual depression, irritability, and anxiety may be related to the elevation of chemicals within the blood system called endorphins. These endorphin levels are higher right before the period and are immediately reduced with the onset of bleeding.

2. Fluid retention. Some findings suggest that many of the characteristics of premenstrual syndrome—abdominal bloating, breast tenderness, and headache—are secondary to an underlying disorder in the endocrine system. For example, altered estrogen levels can induce fluid retention.

3. *Hormonal imbalance.* Studies also show that when estrogen levels are not balanced by other hormones, women can develop fluid retention, breast tenderness, and headaches. The level of another hormone, progesterone, decreases dramatically just before the period, when the PMS symptoms seem to be the worst.

4. *Hypoglycemia.* Many women have twice the concentration of insulin just before their period than what they have during other times of the month. This may account for the fact that PMS women tend to crave sweets during the premenstrual period.

5. *Psychosomatic factors.* Some studies indicate that women with PMS have preexisting problems with anxiety and depression and that these factors may, in fact, trigger the PMS symptoms. This would explain why some women treated with tranquilizers or antidepressants during this period get significant relief.

6. *Vitamin deficiency.* The fluctuations of estrogen prior to your period can cause a deficiency of vitamin B-6 that in turn causes a reduction in the production of the chemical serotonin. Lack of serotonin can contribute to some of the depression. Certain women with PMS have supplemented their diet with vitamin B-6 and have shown significant improvement.

Would changes in my diet make my PMS better?

Dr. Guy E. Abraham is the leader in advocating nutritional therapy for symptoms of premenstrual syndrome. Because of the relationship of certain foods in your diet to the symptoms of PMS, altering what you eat may significantly reduce the problems. Here are some of the recommendations:

- Take a supplement of vitamin B-6 (200 to 800 mg per day) to ease the irritability, tension, bloating, and fatigue. Vitamin E may also relieve some of the breast symptoms.
- Limit the amount of refined sugar, red meat, alcohol, and caffeine you consume. Remember that caffeine is found in coffee, tea, chocolate, and many soft drinks.
- Limit your intake of protein and rely more on fish than red meat protein.
- Limit your daily intake of milk and milk products to 2 servings a day.
- Eat more foods containing an essential fatty acid called linoleic acid (found in safflower oil).

Many women who alter their diets in this way report significant relief from some of the symptoms associated with PMS.

268

What are some other treatments for PMS?

No one really knows exactly why some women with PMS have mild symptoms while others have severe symptoms. Also, since PMS lacks a definite set of criteria for diagnosis, there is no single treatment that will help everyone. However, several categories of treatment, in addition to diet, can be beneficial to some degree.

Exercise and rest. A regular exercise program seems to give relief to many PMS sufferers. Daily exercise not only eases tension but also reduces the amount of fluid you retain. Beginning a regular exercise program and getting an adequate amount of rest are beneficial for your overall health.

Vitamins. As noted before, many physicians recommend that women with PMS take specific vitamin supplements, especially B-6. Remember that vitamins are very complex substances that help your body function, but just because vitamins can help does not mean that *more* vitamins can help *more.* Too much can be dangerous, and you should always check with your physician about dietary supplements.

Water restriction. Because fluid retention and bloating are frequent PMS symptoms, I recommend that women decrease their water intake during the 10 to 14 days before their period. This, combined with less salt intake, can reduce fluid retention and ease the discomfort of bloating.

Nonprescription medications. A variety of different medications for PMS sufferers are available over the counter. Many of these are old standbys, such as acetaminophen, but others are specific products tailored to PMS symptoms. For some women, certain antihistamines can reduce tension and irritability, but any over-the-counter diuretics should be avoided unless cleared by your physician.

Prescription medications. Much of the pain and cramping associated with menstrual periods is caused by chemicals called prostaglandins. Placing women on substances that oppose the prostaglandin activity has significantly helped them. If, as part of your PMS complex of symptoms, you are having severe pain, check with your physician about these medications.

PHYSICAL EXAM

All I generally get during my physical examination is a Pap smear. Should I have a more thorough physical exam?

The answer to this question depends on your age, your previous health history, and your family history. If you are under 40 years of age and in good health, the Pap smear should be your primary concern during your physical examination. However, during that exam, the physician should check your breasts and your blood pressure and make sure that your general health is good.

If you are over 40, especially if you have a family history of hypertension, heart disease, diabetes, or cancer, a more thorough physical examination should be performed. Women over age 40 have an increased risk of heart disease, especially women who smoke. If you fit that category, you should be evaluated just as a man would be for those and other risk factors leading to heart disease. Hypertension often goes undiagnosed in many people simply because their blood pressure has never been checked. A family history of diabetes is reason to check for that disease. After age 40, you should have a thorough physical examination at least every 2 years.

Are my health risks as a woman the same as those for a man my age?

For many years, ailments such as heart disease and lung cancer primarily affected men. But with lifestyle changes and the increased incidence of smoking among women, the risks of heart disease and lung cancer have greatly increased. There is still less chance of developing significant heart disease for you than for a man your age, but you still should have a thorough evaluation.

As women take a more active (and stressful) role in the business world, their health risks are rapidly becoming equal to those of men. Today women live longer than men, but it is predicted that within the next several decades, the differences in life span will begin to narrow.

PAP SMEAR

When should I get my 1st Pap smear?

A woman should receive her 1st Pap smear when she begins to be sexually active. If a woman is not sexually active by age 21, she should begin having yearly Pap smears then.

What is a Pap smear, and why is it important?

Every year, 20,000 cases of cancer of the cervix (the mouth of the uterus) are diagnosed. This type of cancer is curable if it is found early, and the only way to detect it in its early stages is with a simple, painless test called the Pap smear. Named after Dr. George N. Papanicolaou, the physician who invented the test, the Pap smear is a sample of cells collected by the physician who gently inserts a cotton swab into the vaginal opening and scrapes the mouth of the womb.

After these cells are collected, they will be examined under a microscope so that normal cells can be distinguished from abnormal cells and cancer cells. The results of a Pap smear are divided into different classes:

Class I	Normal
Class II	Indicates some degree of inflammation
Class III	Shows abnormal cells but not evidence of cancer
Class IV	Shows cells that strongly suggest cancer
Class V	Shows cells that definitely are cancerous

Depending upon the results, your physician will recommend either treatment or follow-up. Class I Pap smears are reported to the woman as normal, and no treatment or follow-up is necessary. Class II Pap smears may require treatment with a vaginal cream for several weeks, followed by another smear in 3 to 6 months to make sure the condition has not progressed to a higher classification. Class III, IV, and V Pap smears will need definite treatment by a gynecologist.

There has been much debate concerning how often a Pap smear should be performed. Some studies in Canada suggest that for cost effectiveness (the number of positive Pap smears versus the cost), Pap smears probably do not need to be performed every year. My suggestion is that women who have other health risk factors, are sexually active, have had an abnormal Pap smear in the past, or have a family history of cancer of the cervix, uterus, or ovaries should get a Pap smear every year.

VAGINITIS

What are some of the causes of vaginitis?

Vaginitis is an inflammation of the vaginal canal. Its causes range from yeast infections to irritation of the vagina from douches or barrier methods of contraception.

About 75% of all cases of vaginitis are caused by yeast infections, also known as fungal or moniliasis infections, or candidiasis. The symptoms of this type of vaginal infection are intense itching, a cottage-cheeselike discharge, and pain during intercourse. There may also be a rash or redness of the skin outside the vagina that itches or burns.

Yeast vaginitis is caused by an overgrowth of the yeast organisms that inhabit the normal vagina, and it is treated by the insertion into the vagina of a special medication that kills the yeast. Your physician can prescribe this medication and will want to monitor the results.

Why do some women have frequent yeast vaginitis?

There are several causes of frequent bouts of yeast vaginitis, including the following:

- *Tight undergarments or jeans.* Snug-fitting fabrics, especially synthetic fabrics that do not breathe, trap moisture that is conducive to the growth of yeast in the vagina.
- *Diabetes.* The high sugar content of the body fluids of diabetics nourishes infections in the vagina and can cause repeated bouts.
- *Pregnancy.* Pregnant women, perhaps because of hormonal changes, are more susceptible to yeast infections.
- *Antibiotics.* Many antibiotics used for common infections not only cure the infection but also significantly reduce the protective bacteria that live in all women's vaginas. When the protective bacteria are killed, the yeast are not controlled, and overgrowth and infection result.
- *Excessive douching.* Frequent douching can eliminate the normal protective barriers in the vagina as well as cause the vagina to be dry and more susceptible to infection.
- *Hormones.* Women who take hormonal medications, especially birth control pills, are more susceptible to yeast vaginitis.

If I have vaginitis, will my partner catch it during sex?

Generally, no. The yeast organism that causes the vaginitis is difficult to transmit to your sexual partner. Some men, however, will develop a penile irritation or rash reaction to the fungal infection. If this happens, his physician can give him an antibiotic cream at the same time your vaginitis is being treated.

I have a constant vaginal discharge. Is there anything wrong?

Some women have anything from an intermittent to a constant vaginal discharge. Usually, this is a mucus-type discharge that is clear and odorless. Often, the discharge becomes heavier during the middle of the menstrual cycle, probably due to the changes that occur during ovulation.

As long as this vaginal discharge is clear and odorless and is not associated with pain, discomfort, or a bloody component, it is probably quite normal. Women with a profuse, constant discharge should consult their physician to make sure, but be advised that there probably isn't a serious underlying condition.

20.

Problems with the Skin

DRY SKIN

How can I avoid dry skin problems as I get older?

The skin accounts for over 15% of total body weight, and it serves many functions—a protector, an organ of sensation, a regulator of internal temperature, and an eliminator of body waste (sweat). The outer layer of the skin serves as a protective coating while the inner layer provides the support and elasticity we need.

A common concern of adults is dry skin, and there are several things you can do as you grow older to help prevent it. Avoid abrasive facial scrubs and pads. Although removing dead skin can be cosmetically beneficial, it can also destroy the normal skin protection and lead to dry skin and more rapid aging. Also avoid using alcohol on your skin. Alcohol is great for removing excess oil from oily skin, but it can remove too much oil thus drying your skin.

If you have acne, avoid squeezing the pimples or blackheads. Hands off is the general rule because traumatizing your skin in this way can cause injury and scarring.

Even though we love to get out in the sun because it makes us feel and look healthier, sunlight and its ultraviolet rays are major contributors to skin aging. Always use sunscreen when you expect any prolonged exposure.

Exposure to the winter winds and cold weather can also dry the skin. This type of dehydration is a primary cause of future wrinkling.

Suppose I do have very dry skin. Is there anything I can do about it now?

273

The skin seems to become more fragile with age and more easily irritated by chemicals and the air produced by heaters or air conditioners. The body's immune system also seems to lose some of its efficiency as we get older, so the skin is more vulnerable to infection and irritation.

Dermatologists feel that a principal cause of dry skin is an excessive use of soaps and cleansers. It is important to bathe, but it is not necessary to use strong deodorant or heavily perfumed soaps. These soaps should be avoided and replaced by nonirritating natural soaps.

Bathing in very hot water is another cause of skin dehydration. This is especially true in the winter months, when humidity in the air is already very low. Try to bathe in tepid water in all types of weather. Also, using bath oils in the bath water and emollient creams or lotions after your bath can help replace the body's natural oils lost during bathing.

As we get older, many of us are concerned about the fine lines and crow's feet that appear around our eyes. Smokers often have even more pronounced crow's feet and facial wrinkles. Using an eye oil to supermoisturize the very delicate skin around the eyes seems to help.

Stay away from detergent bubble baths and perfumed products. These products, although nice at the time, accelerate the drying effect on the skin.

Always wear loose-fitting clothing. Natural fibers such as cotton breathe and are less irritating to the skin. Some of the more modern fashions seem to depend on synthetic fibers that are tight and binding. Clothing that doesn't let your skin move and breathe freely can increase your chances of skin problems in the future.

Always maintain an adequate fluid intake. It is essential to drink several glasses of water a day not only for your general well-being but also for the health of your skin.

OILY SKIN

Is there anything I can do for very oily skin?

The natural oils in your skin are created by oil glands. When these glands become overactive, an excessive amount of oil is produced creating a bothersome facial condition for many people. External applications of drying lotions can control some of this oil but not all of it. However, the following tips can help:

• Wash with warm water and a nonabrasive soap. Do this any time you feel that your skin is getting greasy.

274

- Avoid brushes and abrasive skin cleaners. They irritate your skin and can cause a swelling or plugging up of the normal oil glands.
- If your skin is exceptionally oily, consult your physician. There are drying agents in the form of soaps that can help control this problem. However, excessive use of these drying soaps or the use of a too-harsh soap can cause burning and redness.

ACNE

What causes acne?

Acne is a skin problem that occurs in over 80% of adolescents and young people. We used to think that acne was caused by dirt and oil on the surface of the skin. We now know that the problem begins deeper, in the sebaceous or oil glands. At puberty, these oil glands begin to produce rather large amounts of a material called sebum. When this sebum cannot pass through the opening of the oil gland (hair follicle), it becomes trapped. The plugged-up gland will then enlarge, forming a kind of pimple, a blackhead. If the duct is completely plugged, a whitehead is formed. The oil inside the pimple attracts bacteria and when the bacteria invade the oil, they create an infection. If the infection continues, the pimple can rupture, forming a cyst. These cysts, or nodules, under the skin are evident in cases of severe acne and can cause severe scarring.

How is acne treated?

The treatment of acne depends upon the severity of the problem. An occasional pimple can be treated with a nonprescription drying agent, such as salicylic acid or benzoyl peroxide.

When acne becomes more widespread, it will require prescription-strength medication—antibiotics and stronger drying agents. If bacteria have invaded the follicles, an antibiotic cream or an oral antibiotic may be necessary. These antibiotics must be taken for a long period of time. A young person placed on antibiotics to help control acne should know that improvement may not be evident for 6 to 8 weeks. The antibiotic therapy will need to be continued for 6 to 12 months.

I've heard that acne can be caused by eating too much chocolate. Is that true?

The many myths regarding the cause of acne have created a great deal of confusion regarding its treatment. The precise cause of acne is still

275

unknown, but it may be due to many factors. Heredity causes some people to have overproductive oil glands, making them more likely to have a blockage of the oil ducts.

Acne is not caused by a failure to clean your face well enough, since pimples start beneath the skin where even the best type of cleaning cannot reach. However, keeping your face clean, especially using drying agents, can remove the excess oil on the skin and open up the oil ducts.

During adolescence, a type of hormone (androgen) is produced that, among other things, stimulates the growth of the oil glands of the skin and triggers the formation of sebum. However, some people with high levels of androgens in their system have no problems with acne while others with normal to low levels of androgens have severe acne. Therefore, it seems that androgens may be connected in some way, but there's no proof that they actually cause acne.

The erroneous belief that acne can be caused by chocolate, greasy french fries, pizza, and the like is probably the most overstated myth. To date, scientists have found no correlation between junk food and the formation of pimples. However, junk food has never been found to be the most nutritious diet, and good nutrition is important for overall health and good, healthy skin.

The last myth regarding acne causes the most confusion among young adolescents. Some people say that sexual activity cures acne while others claim that sex or masturbation can cause it. The truth is that neither of these is correct. Neither sexual activity nor masturbation has any effect on androgen levels, stimulation of the sebaceous glands, or the formation of acne.

Is there any hope for the person with severe acne?

When the sebaceous glands become infected and a cyst is formed, there is a possibility that when the cyst ruptures, it will leave a scar. The large nodules or cysts on the face and the subsequent scar formation can be a very severe and disfiguring disease for many young people.

In the past, not much could be done. However, a new medication on the market may, in certain select cases, provide a great deal of benefit. This medication, isotretinoin, is related to vitamin A and has been used successfully in treating severe acne. A word of caution: This medication has many bothersome side effects, including a dry mouth and lips, irritated eyes, mild nosebleeds, general aches and pains, itching, hair thinning, rash, headaches, and peeling of the palms of the hands and soles of the feet. These side effects are only temporary and do not occur in a lot of people, but isotretinoin is not a medication to be taken lightly.

The exact dose must be carefully controlled by your physician and should be used only for severe cases.

WARTS

What causes warts?

Warts have been with us for centuries. Once thought to be caused by witches' spells or by handling frogs, warts are actually caused by viruses and are some of the most common skin problems physicians treat. The different kinds of warts are caused by different viruses, such as the following:

- The common wart *(verrucca vulgaris)* is a firm, rough, skin-colored elevation of the skin commonly seen on the backs of the hands and the fingers.
- Flat warts *(verruca plana)* are smooth and occur on the face and knees.
- Plantar warts *(verruca plantaris)* occur on the feet and can be very painful.

What are some of the best ways to treat warts?

Treatment of warts is difficult because they are caused by viruses, and as you know, medicine has not found a cure for viruses. Treatment is also complicated by the fact that ⅔ of all warts will probably go away on their own after a period of time.

Here are the most popular methods of treating warts:

1. Applying chemicals such as trichloroacetic acid or salicylic acid. These acids eat away at the warty material on the skin and get down into the bottom part of the wart to kill the virus. These acids should be applied under the direction of a physician, since applying too much, too often can create severe skin reactions.

2. Burning. After a local anesthetic, usually Novocain, has been injected, the wart is actually burned with an electrical charge in a process called electrodessication. This is a relatively painless procedure, except for the injection of the Novocain, and the burned-out area will heal within 2 or 3 weeks.

3. A freezing technique called cryosurgery. Through the use of liquid nitrogen under high pressure, the wart and the underlying tissue are frozen. This freezing causes a blister to form at the base of the wart, which lifts the wart and its viruses away from the skin.

The decision to treat warts really depends on you. If the warts don't hurt and are not disfiguring, leave them alone. Many will go away on their own.

I thought I had something stuck in my foot, but my doctor says I have a wart on my heel.

Plantar warts are very common problems. Because of the extremely sensitive nature of the bottom of the foot, warts there can be quite painful, and you will feel as if you have something stuck in your foot or as if you have a bruise on your foot that hasn't healed.

The complicating factor with plantar warts is that they are more difficult to treat than warts on other parts of the body. The physician will want to take great care and not do anything drastic, since total surgical removal of warts on the bottom of the foot can cause scarring and a very painful foot for the rest of your life.

The best methods to use in taking off plantar warts are cryosurgery and specially applied acids. Cryosurgery, the freezing technique, is relatively painless but must be repeated every 3 to 4 weeks for up to 3 months. Using acids, on the other hand, is often quicker, but does cause a little more pain after application.

PSORIASIS

What is psoriasis, and how can it be treated?

The cells in the epidermis, the outer layer of your skin, normally are shed and replaced in a cycle that takes approximately 4 weeks. New cells originate at the bottom layer of the epidermis, slowly make their way to the top, and are shed. When this process is sped up for unknown reasons, it can be associated with a condition called psoriasis. Characteristics are sharply outlined patches of thickened skin that have a silvery-white scale on them, occurring primarily on the knees and elbows. The scales may cause itching and, when removed, may bleed slightly.

About 2% of the American population has psoriasis, according to the Department of Dermatology, University of Minnesota. The majority develop psoriasis before the age of 30, but childhood psoriasis accounts for about 12% to 15% of all the cases. Psoriasis can affect any age group, and it occurs with equal frequency in males and females.

Psoriasis is a chronic disease. There is no known prevention or cure. The duration of flare-ups can be anywhere from several weeks to many years. Sometimes, the person will have a flare-up that lasts for months, then not have another for several years.

Currently, a treatment for psoriasis is a topical medication. Cortisone creams or ointments have been used with good results. Many times, these cortisone creams are applied and then covered with plastic wrap to increase their penetration deep into the skin.

There is no known connection between psoriasis and cancer, but some anticancer drugs have been found to be effective in its treatment. These are very special and potentially dangerous medications that should be prescribed only under the direction of your physician or dermatologist.

Perhaps the most helpful treatment for psoriasis is the use of ultraviolet light therapy, combined with medication. The treatment, called PUVA, is still considered to be experimental in some institutes but, more and more, qualified physicians are using it.

FUNGAL INFECTION

As I've gotten older, the nails on my big toes have turned yellow. What causes this?

One of my favorite words in medicine is onychomycosis, a very impressive name that simply means a fungal infection under the nails. Your yellow nails are probably caused by onychomycosis. These fungi get into the nail beds and grow, disfiguring and discoloring the nail. When the nail, especially of the great toe, becomes deformed, crooked, and very thickened, the problem is probably caused by onychomycosis.

The difficult part is that this disease is almost totally impossible to cure. Many attempts have been made through using topical creams, removing the nail, and taking oral medications to kill the fungus. The latter is probably the only one that has any real benefit, but the medication is expensive, has some side effects, and must be taken for a long period of time before any results are seen. Even then, there's only a 50–50 chance that medication can help severe onychomycosis. Unless there's a secondary infection or persistent pain, the best thing to do with yellow nails is to leave them alone.

AGE SPOTS

What causes "age spots"?

Age spots are caused by a change in the skin pigmentation or coloring that is part of the normal process of aging. Melanin cells, those that produce a brownish pigment, become overproductive and create a darkening of the area.

Age spots do not turn into cancer. If you do not like them, the best way to prevent them is to take care of your skin throughout your life, especially avoiding excess exposure to sunlight. Many medications sold

279

commercially are supposed to take away age spots, but most of them are ineffective and may cause severe skin allergies. If you are concerned about your age spots, consult your physician before using any medications.

SKIN CANCER

What causes skin cancer?

The most serious consequence of overexposure to the ultraviolet light of the sun is the development of skin cancer. The American Academy of Dermatology reports that most of the 400,000 cases of skin cancer in the United States each year are related to overexposure to the sun. Fortunately, most of these skin cancers, if detected early enough, are treatable and curable.

The American Cancer Society has compiled a list of early warning signs that can help you detect any skin cancer in earlier, more curable stages:

1. A sore that does not heal
2. A change in the size or color of a wart or mole
3. The development of any unusual pigmented area
4. A mole or wart that bleeds

Report any of these early warning signs to your physician. In most cases, you will not have skin cancer, but only a doctor's examination can prove it.

What are some of the types of skin cancer, and how are they treated?

There are 3 major types of skin cancer. Most are caused by overexposure to the ultraviolet light of the sun. A basal cell carcinoma is the most common type and occurs primarily in fair-skinned people. It begins as a small, translucent, pearly, or waxy bump with very tiny blood vessels on its surface and is found mainly on the face, ears, and side of the neck. If treated early by surgical removal, it is nearly 100% curable.

The 2nd most common type is a squamous cell carcinoma. It also occurs primarily in fair-skinned people and is a thick, hard-feeling lesion, which may have a white or yellowish scale. There may also be some skin redness around the lesion. These carcinomas are more difficult to treat than basal cell carcinomas, but if found early enough, they too can be cured.

The 3rd type is the most serious but the least common: malignant melanoma. It starts as a small molelike growth that increases in size, changes color (generally turning dark to black), becomes ulcerated, and bleeds at the slightest touch. Malignant melanomas can spread rapidly to other parts of the body and must be treated immediately with a wide surgical excision. If there is a chance that the malignant melanoma may spread to other parts of the body, the surgeon will recommend that the lymph nodes around the area of the cancer be removed.

SUNBURN

Why does the sun burn our skin?

The light that radiates from the sun is really a spectrum of many different types of rays, the 3 most well-known being ultraviolet, visible light, and infrared light. As light travels from the sun, the ozone layer of the atmosphere absorbs most of the dangerous ultraviolet rays. As it travels further, clouds absorb another 20%, but the remainder of the dangerous ultraviolet light rays gets through. Infrared rays cause us to feel the sun's warmth. Ultraviolet rays, however, do the burning and are more dangerous because you cannot feel them; they cause severe sunburn and skin cancers.

When the sun's ultraviolet rays strike the skin, they begin to damage the cells closest to the top of the skin, causing them to swell. The resulting pain and the redness are caused by the dilation of the blood vessels in the damaged area. In order to protect the skin, the body will form small granules of melanin, a brownish pigment made in specialized skin cells. These cells rise to the surface in response to the ultraviolet radiation. The outcome—a tan—is the body's attempt to save its skin from further damage.

Does the sun hurt some people more than others?

Practically everybody wants a tan in the summer, but the fact remains that too much sun can be painful and dangerous. All of us are at risk from ultraviolet rays, but some people are at much greater risk. People who have blond hair, blue eyes, and light skin that freckles easily run the greatest risk of developing skin cancers. People with Irish and Scottish heritage are also much more likely to burn and not tan. The reason is that through the generations very few melanin pigments have remained under the skin's surface that could create a tan, thus protecting the skin.

How can I avoid getting a sunburn?

We all know that the sun's ultraviolet rays can be harmful, but it is almost impossible to enjoy the summer without getting out in those rays. So let's look at some tips for protecting yourself from the damage the sun can do.

1. Gradually build up your exposure to the sun. Never start by trying to get a tan in the middle of the day. Go out the 1st 3 or 4 days for only 10 to 15 minutes at a time in the early morning and the late afternoon. Over a period of several weeks, gradually increase the amount of time exposure you have to the sun.

2. Avoid the sun altogether between 10:00 A.M. and 2:00 P.M. These are the hours that the sun and the ultraviolet rays are at their strongest.

3. Use a sunscreen with a sun protection factor recommended by your doctor and use it properly.

4. Remember that you can burn even on cool, cloudy days. Watch out for the wind because it gives you a false sense of coolness while you burn your skin.

5. Finally, some drugs you take, such as antibiotics, can increase your chance of burning. If you are on any medication, check with your doctor to see if your medicine could affect your exposure to the sun.

If I do get a sunburn, what's the best way to treat it?

Perhaps the worst feeling in the world is to be on a long-awaited vacation and end up in your hotel room looking like a lobster and feeling terrible. Mild sunburns generally respond to measures that hydrate (increase the water content of) the skin. Swelling, redness, and heat can be relieved by applying cold compresses. Application of plain petroleum jelly, a steroid cream, or a steroid spray can provide further relief. Check the drugstore for water-based preparations that also may be of some benefit. Regular doses of aspirin can also significantly relieve discomfort.

If the sunburn is severe enough to cause blisters, especially over a large part of the body, you may benefit from a short course of steroids. Because a blistered sunburn is deeper, it is much more painful and often requires codeine or other more potent narcotics for relief of pain.

Severe generalized sun reactions should be treated as any 2nd- or 3rd-degree burn of the skin. With widespread burns, you may need to be placed on intravenous fluids because the burned skin will seep and lose a tremendous amount of internal liquid. The presence of blisters and raw areas increases the potential of infection, so treatment will include antibiotics and creams to prevent infection and scarring.

What are sunscreens and who should use them?

Let's take the 2nd part of the question 1st and say that all people should use some form of sunscreen when they are exposed to long periods of sunlight. The purpose of a sunscreen is to provide a film or coating over the skin that adds extra protection in blocking out the dangerous and damaging ultraviolet rays of the sun. Several chemicals within sunscreens accomplish this task, but the most common is para-aminobenzoic acid (PABA). The main difference between suntan lotions and sunscreens is that the sunscreen has PABA and helps protect the skin from ultraviolet damage. Lotions increase exposure.

All sunscreens are required to specify how much of the sun they block out. This is referred to as the sun protection factor, or SPF. The SPF values range from 1 to 15 or higher; the smaller numbers give the least protection, and the larger numbers the greatest protection.

Ideally, a person who is highly susceptible to sunburn or who will be out in the sun for long periods of time should use a high SPF sunscreen. It may be possible as the skin begins to tan naturally to lower the number of the sunscreen.

Sunscreens are highly effective in preventing sunburn, but they must be used properly. Almost all sunscreens wash off immediately with excess moisture, such as sweating or swimming and, unlike many suntan lotions, have to be reapplied almost constantly.

What are some of the medications that can increase my sensitivity to the sun?

Many of the common medications you take for infections, high blood pressure, diabetes, and other conditions can increase your sensitivity to the sun.

Antibiotics, such as sulfa and tetracycline, increase your sensitivity, as do tranquilizers and diuretics.

Oral contraceptives have been associated with increased pigmentation, a condition referred to as chloasma, in women exposed to the sun. It has also been found that certain antiseptics found in soaps, detergents, or cosmetics can also increase sensitivity to the sun. Perfumes are frequent culprits.

Ask your doctor if any medication you're taking may make you more sensitive to the sun. Chances are, if your medicine makes you more sensitive, you'll need to stay out of the sun or take extra precautions.

Are tanning centers dangerous?

Yes. These centers use bulbs that emit ultraviolet light but little heat. Such radiation can cause degenerative changes of the skin, wrinkling, color spots, and other cosmetic problems. Exposure to ultraviolet light used in tanning centers may also cause a photosensitivity in many people who are taking the drugs that we talked about before. And, of course, the evidence linking solar radiation to skin cancer is well established.

In spite of these facts, indoor tanning centers have recently become very popular. Since this tanning takes place in air-conditioned booths in a fraction of the time it takes to get a tan in normal sunlight, these centers attract millions of Americans who want an "instant" tan.

Everyone should be cautious in utilizing tanning centers. If you "must" use them, make sure that you use proper eye protection (ultraviolet reflecting goggles) and expose your body to the ultraviolet light for only short periods of time. The same precautions for sun tanning centers must be observed as for the sun at the beach. People with fair complexions, known sensitivity or burning potential, or a family history of skin cancer should use tanning centers with great caution or, preferably, not at all.

PRURITUS

What causes my skin to itch?

Pruritus, the severe itching of undamaged skin, is a common problem for many adults. Usually limited to certain areas, such as behind the ears or on the hands, ankles, or wrists, it often occurs because of stress, much like headaches or stomach problems. Cold, wet compresses can help relieve itching, as can the addition of proper moisturizers to the skin.

A frequent cause of itching, especially in older people, is dry skin. Decreasing the number of baths you take per week and increasing the use of moisturizers can relieve some of this itching. Generalized itching over the entire body can be a sign of certain diseases, such as diabetes, thyroid disease, or gout. If you have unexplainable itching that persists more than a week or so, consult your physician.

ECZEMA

What is eczema?

Eczema is simply an inflammation of the skin. It can occur on any part of the body, is manifested by red, irritated, oozing patches, and can be caused by anything from contact with certain types of plants (poison ivy) to skin infections or allergies.

Most cases of eczema can be controlled with the application of topical cortisone creams. These creams will relieve the allergic reaction to the skin and prevent further oozing. However, people with eczema must be cautious because the lesions can become infected and drain yellowish, infected material. If this occurs, special antibiotic ointments or tablets must be taken before the eczema will clear.

SCABIES

What is scabies?

Scabies is a skin disease caused by the organism *Sarcoptes scabiei*. The disease has plagued people for thousands of years, but it became quite well known during World Wars I and II when it contributed to what was called the camp itch. Scabies outbreaks occur in cycles, and once it was felt that the cycles contributed to the well-known 7-year itch.

Scabies is becoming more prevalent in our society today and along with its increased occurrence comes a great deal of misunderstanding. Many people think that scabies is an infection, which means they are unclean, or that it is like having a sexually transmitted disease.

If your doctor tells you that you have scabies, don't be embarrassed. It's a common condition seen in all socioeconomic levels of society. It doesn't mean that you are unclean, just that you've come in contact with the scabies mite.

Scabies spreads by direct contact with someone who has been infected: children holding hands when they play games; people sharing clothes, or sleeping in the same bed with someone who has scabies. Scabies mites do not, however, jump from person to person, and scabies cannot be contracted simply by being around someone with the problem.

What happens when I get scabies?

When you come into contact with the scabies organism, it burrows and lives under your skin where the female mite lays several eggs each day. The eggs hatch, and the mites travel to the surface of the skin.

It is extremely difficult to see the female scabies mite without the aid of a magnifying glass, but the results of her burrowing can be seen on the skin as zigzag crevices—greyish-white threads on the skin's surface that mark her trail. If your doctor believes that you have scabies, he or she will take a small portion of 1 of these burrows and examine it under the microscope to identify the scabies mite.

How is scabies treated?

The treatment for scabies is very effective and easy. It consists of applying a lotion that kills the scabies mite. You apply this lotion over your entire body at night and wash it off thoroughly in the morning for approximately 3 days. This kills the scabies mite under the skin and relieves the itching. However, there may be some degree of itching up to 2 to 3 weeks afterward, even though the scabies mite has been destroyed. Scabies in pregnant women and children under 6 should be treated by a physician.

RINGWORM

What is ringworm and how can it be treated?

Ringworm is actually a superficial infection of the skin caused by a fungus. (Because of the way it looks, it was once believed that ringworm was caused by a small worm that crawled under the skin and formed a circular patch.) These fungal infections can invade the scalp, the body, the feet, the hands, the nails, or the groin, and they are caused by 3 different types of fungi: Microsporum, Trichophyton, and Epidermophyton. Collectively, they are known as ringworm.

Ringworm has a characteristic appearance on the body—a circular, reddened, raised area with a light area in the center. The raised area can have small blisters on it and may be scaly. When ringworm occurs on the scalp or the groin, there can be a loss of hair around the infection.

When ringworm becomes inflamed, it can itch and be irritated and sore. In its chronic phase, often between the toes, it has much less inflammation but a great deal of itching.

Ringworm, because it is caused by a fungus, is treated by a specific antifungal medication. If you think that you have ringworm, consult your physician for the proper medication.

CONTACT DERMATITIS

What is contact dermatitis?

Contact dermatitis is a particular type of skin inflammation caused by contact with substances found in the everyday environment. The inflammation of dermatitis appears as redness, swelling, itching, or blistering. In severe cases, there is a great deal of pain. Inflammation can also be associated with the secondary bacterial infection, causing oozing of yellowish material.

The primary treatment of dermatitis is to control the inflammation, usually through the use of topical cortisone creams that reduce the inflammation and allow the underlying skin to heal. The 2nd part of the treatment is to identify the specific substance within the environment that causes this reaction. Once this substance has been identified, it must be avoided in the future.

Anyone can get dermatitis. However, the people who are at greater risk are those who have the most constant exposure. Housewives, for instance, frequently get dermatitis from soaps, detergents, cleaning fluids, sprays, and other irritating materials used around the house. Industrial workers commonly get dermatitis from constant exposure to industrial chemicals on the job.

Dermatitis can also be caused by cosmetics, hair sprays, deodorants, the nickel in watches, the leather in shoes, and many other everyday substances.

The most common cause of contact dermatitis in the United States is a plant—poison ivy, and its relatives, poison oak and sumac.

POISON IVY

How do I identify poison ivy?

Always remember the saying, "Leaves 3, let it be." Poison ivy is a pretty green plant that has 3 leaves on the end of the stalk, with the stem of the central leaflet growing longer than the stem of the 2 leaflets on the side. It grows as a low plant, shrub, or climbing vine, and during certain periods of the year, it has yellow-green flowers and whitish berries. Poison ivy leaves are shiny when they first come out, and they turn red and yellow in autumn. If you have any doubt, don't touch it.

What is it about poison ivy that causes contact dermatitis?

People who are allergic to poison ivy are actually allergic to the oil in the plant itself. Once the oil gets on the skin it causes a severe inflammation of that portion of the skin. This inflammation generally begins as itching and after 2 to 3 days progresses into a red, swollen area with blisters. When you scratch it, the poison ivy oil will spread up the scratch and cause the blistering and redness to spread. This is a characteristic of poison ivy that is not typical of other types of contact dermatitis.

If you have been exposed to poison ivy, *immediately* wash the contact areas thoroughly with soap and water to remove all of the plant's oily residue. If, after several days, you do develop some redness and itching in those areas, immediately apply some over-the-counter hydrocortisone cream which will reduce the inflammation. If the inflammation continues or begins to spread, contact your physician for stronger hydrocortisone cream. If the inflammation becomes severe enough, you may need cortisone shots or tablets to reduce the inflammation. And don't scratch.

21.

Understanding Blood Sugar
and the Thyroid

DIABETES

What is diabetes?

Over 2000 years ago, Hippocrates described a condition in which the urine contained excessive amounts of sugar, causing it to have a peculiar odor. In fact, he called it the sweet urine disease. The condition Hippocrates was referring to was diabetes, and the same description holds true today. However, much knowledge has been gained about what diabetes is and how to treat it.

Diabetes is a complex disease, but in simple terms it means that an excessive amount of sugar accumulates in the blood and the urine. Sugar, or glucose, is the body's main source of energy, and it is utilized by every cell of the body. When we eat food that contains sugar, the sugar is immediately absorbed through the lining of the digestive tract and accumulates within the blood. The blood sugar is then transported to every cell of the body by a substance called insulin.

Insulin is produced by a gland called the pancreas that sits in the upper middle portion of your abdomen, close to the stomach. In a person with diabetes, the production of insulin is nonexistent or insufficient, or the body is unable to utilize it properly. Because there is not enough insulin to carry the sugar from the blood into the cells, the sugar accumulates in the blood. Sugar is normally found in the blood in small amounts to maintain energy levels in the cells of the body. However, for diabetics, the sugar level in the blood rises so high, that it must

288

be excreted by the kidneys. The urine, therefore, will have a high level of sugar.

Are all diabetics alike?

No. There are basically 2 different types of individuals who have diabetes. The 1st type includes people born with a total lack of insulin in the pancreas. They are known as juvenile or Type I diabetics because the symptoms of diabetes show up at an early age. In the second type of diabetic, diabetes occurs later in life, not because of a total lack of insulin but because of an insufficient amount of it. This is called adult onset or Type II diabetes.

Dividing diabetes into these 2 categories has more significance than mere nomenclature—it explains why some diabetics have to take insulin and others can control their condition with diet or oral medication. Because of the absence of insulin, Type I diabetics almost always have to be on insulin shots. Type II diabetics, the people who have some insulin but not enough, can usually control their diets or take oral medication and maintain normal health without insulin injections.

What are some of the more common symptoms of diabetes?

Not all people with diabetes have symptoms. Some people discover the condition only when their urine or blood is tested. Even when diabetic symptoms are present, they vary from person to person in type and intensity. But there are some common symptoms that *could* indicate the presence of diabetes:

Frequent urination. In diabetes, when the blood sugar level rises, large amounts of water have to be retained within the system to neutralize the high sugar content. This would cause the diabetic to constantly produce more urine and need to urinate frequently.

Intense thirst. To maintain this high production of urine caused by elevated blood sugar, the body will signal the need for large fluid intake to counteract the loss of urine—thirst.

Rapid loss of weight and extreme hunger. Because the undiagnosed diabetic can't utilize the sugar within the blood, the body must draw its energy from stored fat and protein. The body will actually eat away at its normal reserves, causing rapid weight loss and triggering intense hunger.

Feelings of fatigue. Our energy levels are maintained when the body can properly utilize sugar. In diabetes, this does not occur, so that the diabetic will often complain of being tired and will easily become fatigued.

Other symptoms that can go along with diabetes are *blurred vision, slow healing of cuts, persistent itching* or *skin rashes, nausea, frequent vaginal infections,* and *dizziness.*

If you have any of these symptoms, it does not mean that you have diabetes. However, if you have a family history of diabetes, are overweight, or are not feeling up to par, you should consult your physician to make sure you are not 1 of the millions of Americans with undiagnosed diabetes.

Why do some diabetics go into a coma?

Because of the deficiency of insulin, a diabetic's cells are unable to obtain enough glucose for energy. Therefore, the body has to turn to its supply of fat tissue for this energy. Fat is a good fuel because it yields about twice as many calories per ounce as sugar, but when the body uses fat for energy, certain chemicals called ketones and ketoacids are formed as byproducts. (Ketoacids cause the "fruity" odor in the breath of a severe diabetic.) As these chemicals accumulate, they cause the blood to become very acid, and a condition called acidosis develops. When acidosis reaches a certain point, a person can go into a diabetic coma. Diabetic coma occurs primarily in people with Type I diabetes and is rare in people who have Type II diabetes.

Are some people more prone to diabetes than others?

The primary factor in determining who will or will not develop diabetes is heredity; people with diabetic parents or close relatives are predisposed to developing diabetes. If your mother or father is diabetic, and especially if insulin is required for treatment, you stand a 50% chance of developing the disease.

In addition to heredity, other factors play an important role in determining who will develop diabetes. These factors include obesity, pregnancy, chronic diseases of the liver, chronic infections of the pancreas, and certain viral infections.

Of course, some people develop diabetes for no apparent reason. That's why it's so important to watch for warning signs that indicate the possibility of the disease. If you have any of the warning signs, a family history of diabetes, or are more than 20 pounds overweight, you should check with your physician periodically to make sure that your blood sugar is normal.

How can my doctor find out if I have diabetes?

The 2 basic tests used to diagnose diabetes detect the sugar content of the blood and the urine. If your physician suspects that you may be at risk of developing diabetes, he or she will order a blood sugar test. A random blood sugar count above 160 to 180 indicates diabetes, and no further testing needs to be done. However, in many people suspected of having diabetes, the random blood sugar is normal. If this is the case, the physician may test the blood sugar 2 hours after the individual eats a lot of sugar with a heavy meal. This is a 2-hour postprandial blood sugar. If this count is above 160, the diagnosis of diabetes is made. These tests are coordinated with urine specimens collected at the same time to see if sugar is present in the urine.

A more definitive test is the glucose tolerance test. A person who has been fasting is given a predetermined amount of sugar in a very sweet drink. Over the next 3 hours, the urine and the blood are tested. Any person's blood sugar will rise in response to this drink, but a diabetic will far exceed the limits, and the diagnosis can then be made.

If I have diabetes, will I have to take insulin?

It depends. Type I, or juvenile, diabetics will have to be on insulin injections because they simply do not have any insulin. Some Type II, or adult onset, diabetics will need shots, also. But the vast majority of diabetics in the Type II category will *not* need insulin injections because their condition can be controlled by other means.

The 1st approach is to help the Type II diabetic achieve ideal body weight, according to age, height, and body structure. When you have diabetes, the closer you are to your ideal weight, the easier it is to control the disease. An ADA (American Diabetes Association) diet is specifically modified to allow the diabetic to take in an appropriate amount of calories for weight reduction *and* for regulation of the energy supply. Regardless of the other treatments you need, following this specific diet is critical to present and future control of diabetes.

After you have reached you ideal weight, if your blood sugar is still not in the normal range, your doctor will probably place you on oral medication. The basic premise of the pills is to help "pump up" your pancreas to produce more insulin and increase the effectiveness that insulin has within your body.

Exercise is also a critical part of the treatment for 2 reasons: it helps control your blood sugar, and it helps you achieve your ideal body weight. Exercise also increases the effectiveness of many of the medications used for diabetes.

The treatment for the diabetic is tailored to each individual's specific needs, and it is mandatory that patient, doctor, and staff work together for the success of this program.

Why all the fuss about diabetes? Is it really that important to control?

Diabetes is a leading cause of blindness, heart disease, and kidney failure. Diabetes, if left uncontrolled, can also cause impotence, increased incidence of infection, loss of limbs due to gangrene, and ataxia, a nervous disorder that causes loss of muscle coordination. Uncontrolled diabetes, directly or indirectly, is a leading cause of death in this country. So, you can see that diabetes is not a disease that should be ignored. Diabetes that is brought under better control is less likely to cause these complications.

Is low blood sugar the same thing as diabetes?

No. When your blood sugar is too low, the condition is called hypoglycemia. Diabetes means that your blood sugar is too high.

In the past few years, hypoglycemia has become a sort of fashionable condition, and it has been blamed for fatigue, weak spells, craving of sweets, and weight gain. In true hypoglycemia, the body has an unusual reaction to the ingestion of sugar. Normally, when we eat sugar, the blood sugar will rise to a certain point (but not as high as a diabetic's) and then fall back down to a *normal* range within an hour or so. People with hypoglycemia respond to the intake of sugar just as a normal person, but within 1 to 2 hours, their blood sugar will drop very low. When the blood sugar reaches its lowest point the symptoms of hypoglycemia occur.

All parts of the body, including the brain, require energy from sugar. When the sugar level drops too low, symptoms such as trembling, hunger, sweating, headache, nausea, drowsiness, dizziness, blurred vision, and tingling sensations occur. In a typical hypoglycemic reaction, you feel fine just after eating a fairly good meal. But a couple of hours later, you feel as if the plug has been pulled and all your energy has drained. You may sweat and feel trembly, fatigued, and faint. The immediate response is to eat a candy bar. Sure enough, within several minutes you feel better, but an hour or 2 later, the symptoms recur. It would seem logical that when your blood sugar drops too low, you should take in more sugar. Logical, yes, but it doesn't work because the hypoglycemic's reaction to sugar is abnormal. Just like diabetics, hypoglycemics should be placed on diets that are low in sugar. Most hypoglycemics find that eating high-protein midmorning, midafternoon, and bedtime snacks also helps maintain a normal blood sugar level.

292

HYPERTHYROIDISM AND HYPOTHYROIDISM

What does my thyroid gland do?

The thyroid gland is situated in your neck right below your Adam's apple and has 2 parts, 1 on each side of the front of the neck. These 2 lobes are connected with a small piece of tissue called the isthmus.

The thyroid gland produces the thyroid hormone that helps regulate your weight, heart rate, bowels, skin (such as the release of melanin to the cells for protection from the sun's harmful rays), and nervous system. When problems occur within the thyroid, the symptoms can spread throughout the body.

A specific problem you can have is the production of too much thyroid hormone—hyperthyroidism. A person with this condition will have increased body metabolism causing weight loss, trembling, fast heart rate, constipation, and a sensitivity to hot weather.

If you do not produce enough of the thyroid hormone (hypothyroidism), many of the reverse symptoms can occur, including rapid weight gain, increased fatigue, slow heart rate, sluggishness, and a decrease in the ability to concentrate.

Fortunately, both conditions are treatable.

How are these thyroid problems treated?

If you have the symptoms of hypothyroidism, your physician will want to confirm the diagnosis with a simple blood test that will show whether or not you are producing enough thyroid hormone. In the vast majority of the cases of hypothyroidism, the thyroid gland simply fails to produce enough chemical. Treatment of hypothyroidism consists of placing the individual on thyroid hormone supplements, usually pills, to regulate the amount of thyroid hormone in the body. If your physician places you on thyroid supplements, make sure you take them exactly as directed. Overmedication can make your thyroid level too high and can mimic the symptoms of hyperthyroidism.

If your physician finds that your thyroid gland produces too much hormone, hyperthyroidism, there are several options for treatment. In some people, the thyroid gland is treated with a safe level of radiation, called I-131, that will destroy the parts of the thyroid gland that overproduce. Other people can be treated with medications that block production of the thyroid hormone. Finally, people with hyperthyroidism not treatable with the other methods will have to undergo surgery to remove all or part of the thyroid gland.

293

Even if my thyroid is normal, can I take the hormone to help me lose weight?

No. It was fairly common practice in the past to give obese people a thyroid hormone to increase their metabolic rate and thus decrease their weight. If you have a normal level of thyroid hormone, tampering with that level—taking thyroid hormone when you do not really need it—can cause more problems than benefits. Never take thyroid hormone unless tests confirm that your thyroid level is not normal. Taking a friend's thyroid medication, or any other prescription medication, can be potentially dangerous.

22.

Cancer

ABNORMAL CELL GROWTH

What is cancer?

Cancer is a group of many different types of diseases that affects the body's cells. Cells are the tiny building blocks that make up all the different parts of the body—skin, lungs, bones, digestive tract—and all these cells are in a constant state of change. The cells grow, mature, die, and are almost immediately replaced with new cells.

During cell growth, 1 cell splits and becomes 2 new cells. This process is continued until millions of cells are formed into skin, muscle, or brain tissue.

If the cells divide without any order, a growth known as a tumor begins. A tumor may be benign (not cancerous) or malignant (cancerous).

With cancer, something has gone wrong with the normal growth of a cell. When normal growth is altered, the cell divides abnormally, at a faster rate, and can spread. These cells do not function like regular cells, and they crowd out the healthy cells that keep the body going.

CAUSES

Can almost anything cause cancer?

The statement that "everything causes cancer" is a myth not founded on scientific fact. Actually, there are relatively few causes of the abnormal cell growth we call cancer, mainly repeated contact of the cell with substances known as carcinogens. These carcinogens are materials that

295

seem to cause the disorderly cell division resulting in cancer. Known carcinogens include tobacco smoke, sunlight, x-rays, and certain chemicals.

Scientists also suspect that some people are more likely than others to develop cancer, but the specific reasons are as yet unknown.

What are the most frequent types of cancer in men and in women?

In men, lung cancer occurs most frequently, followed closely by colon cancer, then prostate and rectal cancer.

In women, breast and lung cancer are the most common, followed by colon and rectal cancer, and cancer of the uterus. Actual percentages of deaths attributable to cancer are as follows:

	Type	Percentage of Deaths
MEN	lung	35
	colon	12
	prostate	10

	Type	Percentage of Deaths
WOMEN	breast	18
	lung	18
	colon	15

EARLY DETECTION

Why is early detection so important?

Of the 400,000 cancer deaths in the United States each year, the American Cancer Society says that 200,000 could be prevented by early detection and treatment. For the 12 most common cancers that cause over 300,000 deaths, the long-term survival rate of people with localized disease is *80%* greater than those in whom the disease has spread or metastasized. Almost all cancer experts agree that when the growth of the cancer is still localized and has not spread, there's a high probability of cure. If you have cancer, early detection provides greater hope for cure.

How can I recognize cancer in my body?

The 2 strongest recommendations for fighting cancer today are to (1) stop smoking and (2) regularly look for early warning signs or symptoms of cancer and bring them to the attention of your doctor.

Everyone should memorize and thoroughly understand the 7 warning signs of cancer:

1. A change in your bowel or bladder habits may signify colon, prostate, or bladder cancer.
2. A sore that does not heal, especially on the mouth, lip, tongue, or skin, may indicate oral or skin cancer.
3. Any unusual rectal or vaginal bleeding or vomiting of blood should be reported to your physician immediately. Colon cancers, uterine cancers, and cancers of the digestive system can cause these symptoms.
4. Take note of a thickening or lump in the breast, armpit, groin, or elsewhere. Small or large, hard or soft, a lump under the skin or in the breast should be reported to your physician.
5. Persistent indigestion and difficulty in swallowing can be early warning signs of cancer of the esophagus or stomach.
6. An obvious change in a mole or wart—a darkening in color, a loss of color, an increase in size, or bleeding—may indicate skin cancer.
7. A nagging, persistent cough or hoarseness, especially accompanied by coughing up blood, may indicate the presence of lung cancer.

At the first sign of any of these symptoms, you should immediately consult your physician. It does not mean you have cancer, but it does mean that the cause of the symptom needs to be investigated. Remember, the key words are *early detection.*

How often should I get examined to detect cancer early?

There is a set of basic guidelines for the kinds and frequency of early detection exams. Here are the recommendations approved by the American Cancer Society:

Test	Patient Age	Frequency
Breast self-examination	Over 20	Monthly
Breast examination by physician	20–40	Every 3 years
Breast examination by physician	40+	Annually
Digital rectal examination	40+	Annually

Test	Patient Age	Frequency
Stool checked for blood	40+	Annually
Mammography	35–40	1 baseline study
Mammography	40–49	Every 1–2 years
Mammography	50+	Annually
Pap smear	20–65 and sexually active teenagers	2 normal consecutive smears 1 year apart, then every 3 years
Pap smear	After menopause	Annually
Sigmoidoscopy	Over 50	Every 3–5 years

These should be used as basic guidelines and do not apply for people in a high-risk category. Consult your physician regarding more specific guidelines or exceptions.

WHO GETS CANCER?

Can you inherit cancer?

Since cancer happens so often, many families will have several affected members. Most of the time, these different types of cancer that occur within families are just chance or are associated with a specific factor such as smoking, occupation, or diet. However, studies show that close relatives of people who have cancer of the breast, stomach, colon, lung, and uterus are more likely that other people to develop these cancers themselves.

There is no single explanation for this fact. Common lifestyles may be a factor. Genetics may also be a part, but as yet, there is no proof that cancer is inherited.

What are my chances of developing cancer?

The American Cancer Society states that this depends a lot on your sex, age, and family history. Over 800,000 people will develop cancer within the next year; cancer will affect 1 in every 4 people and 2 out of every 3 families.

Age is the overriding risk factor for development of cancer. With every 10-year increase after the age of 25, there is a doubling of the incidence of cancer, and people over 65 years of age have a much greater chance of dying of the disease.

In some specific cancers, a family history is extremely important. For women, if their mother or sister developed breast cancer, they have a far greater risk of developing breast cancer than women with no breast cancer in their family.

Lifestyles are another extremely important factor. People who smoke, drink excessive amounts of alcohol, and are frequently overexposed to sunlight are much more susceptible to developing particular types of cancer. Cigarette smoking is a causative factor in lung, bladder, mouth, larynx, pancreas, and possibly kidney cancer. Alcohol may be a causative agent in the formation of cancers of the mouth, throat, esophagus, and liver. Occupation is responsible for less than 5% of all cancers in the United States, but particular occupations can greatly increase the incidence of cancer. For example, asbestos workers have a higher incidence of a particular type of lung cancer.

Does race make any difference in the incidence of cancer?

Black males have a higher rate of cancer than other groups in this country, especially in the development of lung, prostate, and colon cancer after age 40.

Black females also have a higher rate of large bowel cancer and should be especially alert to the early warning signs and early detection of colon cancer. Uterine and breast cancer are also found more frequently among black females.

SURVIVAL RATE

If I develop cancer, what are my chances of survival?

Today, the chances of surviving cancer are better than ever before. With early detection and proper treatment, many people can not only live healthy, productive lives, but they can actually be cured of their cancer. (A person is considered cured after 5 years with no recurrence or evidence of the disease.)

For example, the 5-year survival rate for people with cancer of the uterus has risen to 81%. That means 5 years after the detection of cancer in the uterus, 81% of these women will still be alive. For cancer of the breast, the rate is 74%; prostate cancer, 68%; colon cancer, 49%; and rectal cancer, 48%.

The most dramatic changes have occurred in the treatment of different cancers of children. Childhood cancers such as certain leukemia, cancer of the bone and kidney, and Hodgkin's disease are potentially curable in many children.

Cancer that is detected, and detected early, can be treated and its victims can still lead full, normal lives. There are more than 3 million

Americans alive today who have had cancer. About 2 million of them have already survived 5 years or more.

The best way to survive cancer is to begin lifestyle changes that can dramatically reduce your chances of developing it. In addition, begin an early detection program based on the 7 warning signs of cancer and have frequent checkups with your physician, especially if you are in a high-risk category.

TYPES

Are all cancers alike?

Almost all types of cancer are different, depending upon the type of cell that creates the cancer and the part of the body it invades. Breast cancer is an entirely different disease from prostate cancer. Prostate cancer is entirely different from skin cancer. Even though the cells are cancerous, their characteristics, ability to spread to other parts of the body, and treatment are very different.

How a physician assesses a particular cancer depends on the site of the body it invades, the type of cell, and the depth or extent to which the cancer has spread. These criteria and others are utilized by your physician and a cancer specialist to determine recommendations for treatment.

The treatments for cancer vary like the cancers themselves. Many cancers respond dramatically to surgery. Others respond better to the use of medications (chemotherapy), and others respond to radiation treatment. Not all cancers are alike, but all cancers are serious.

How common is skin cancer?

Skin cancer is quite common, but because of its high degree of early diagnosis, the cure rate is good. With the exception of malignant melanoma, a rare type of skin cancer, the overall cure rate for skin cancers is 90%.

Most skin growths are noncancerous, but any new growth or a sore that does not heal should be brought to the attention of your physician.

How is cancer of the prostate detected?

The symptoms of prostatic cancer are often the same as those of a man whose prostate is simply enlarged—a change in the ability to urinate, difficulty controlling the force or flow of the stream, having to get up frequently to urinate at night, or the development of traces of blood in the urine. However, cancer of the prostate is best detected through an annual rectal examination; in this way, the physician can directly examine the prostate and detect any unusual enlargements or nodules. If any are found, they can be biopsied (a portion taken and examined under a microscope) for a definite diagnosis.

How can cancer of the colon be detected?

More than 100,000 new cases of cancer of the colon are detected each year; 90% in men and women over the age of 40. You may be at higher risk of colon cancer if you have other problems in your digestive tract, such as chronic ulcerative colitis or congenital multiple polyposis. Diets that are high in fat or low in fiber may also increase your chance of developing colon cancer.

The symptoms of colon cancer include a change in your bowel habits, bright red or black blood in your stools, or persistent abdominal discomfort, gas, or pain.

Because blood is usually passed in the stool of people with undetected colon cancer, checking for this blood is an easy screening test. Called the Hemoccult Test, it is available at your local pharmacy or from your physician. If you are over 40, your physician should perform an annual digital rectal examination, and if you're over 44, your physician will probably recommend a special test called a proctosigmoidoscopy. In this examination, your physician can take a look deep inside the intestine through a small tube inserted through the rectum, then 12″ to 16″ into the colon. This uncomfortable, but relatively painless test, greatly increases the chances of early cancer detection.

How common is breast cancer?

Approximately 1 out of every 11 American women will get breast cancer at some time in her life. It is the major killer of women in their 40's and the leading cause of cancer in all women. These factors are extremely disturbing, especially knowing that most breast cancers, if discovered early enough, can be treated and even cured.

Breast cancer usually appears as a painless lump or thickening in the breast, most frequently in the upper outer portion of the breast. From there, if left untreated, it can spread to the lymph nodes in the armpit and to other parts of the body. Other changes that may indicate breast cancer include a persistent swelling, a dimpling of the skin, redness, skin irritation, pain, or tenderness.

Breast self-examination is *the most* important test that a woman can perform during her lifetime. Simple and easy to learn, this examination allows a woman to check her breasts, every month, for any of the above

301

changes. If they are found, she can immediately report them to her physician for a more thorough evaluation.

DIET

Can diet affect my chances of developing cancer?

Current evidence suggests that many common cancers are influenced by diet. Although the exact contribution of diet cannot be determined, there are several important dietary guidelines designed to reduce your risk of developing cancer:

- Eat less foods high in saturated and unsaturated fats. Fats in your diet should be reduced to approximately 30% of your daily calories. The major sources of fat in the American diet are fatty meats, whole milk and dairy products, and cooking oils.
- Eat fruits, vegetables, and whole-grain cereals daily, especially those high in vitamin C and vitamin A.
- Eat very little salt-cured, salt-pickled, or smoked food.
- Drink alcohol only in moderation.
- Increase your consumption of fiber from foods such as fruits and vegetables and whole-grain cereals.

TREATMENT

How is cancer treated?

The treatment of cancer depends upon the age of the patient, the site of the cancer, and the type of cell that has caused the cancer. Basically, however, there are 3 principal modes of cancer therapy. The surgical procedure is directed at the total removal of all the cancer cells, the theory being that once the cancer cells have been removed, there is no chance that they can spread to other parts of the body. An example of surgical treatment of cancer is mastectomy in which all or a portion of the cancerous breast is removed.

A 2nd treatment is the use of radiation. This has been highly effective in treating certain types of cancer and is used in place of, or in conjunction with, surgery to destroy the cancer or inhibit its growth.

The 3rd form of therapy is the use of special medications—chemotherapy. This treatment is feared by most people because of its side effects, but it is highly effective alone or in conjunction with radiation or surgery.

A cancer specialist (oncologist) will review your specific type of cancer and recommend, along with your personal physician, the type of therapy best suited to your needs. This discussion should include choices of treatment and the possible side effects.

23.

Anxiety and Depression

ANXIETY

My doctor says that I am suffering from anxiety. What could be causing it?

Some anxiety, or a feeling of nervous tension, is normal and even beneficial during times of extreme stress or danger. For instance, if you have just been laid off from work, some anxiety may create the motivation you need to seek another job. However, many people suffer from this feeling of extreme nervous tension for no real reason. In such individuals, the anxiety is exaggerated and may be accompanied by feelings of depression, doom, or fear that they are going to lose control or "go mad." This kind of anxiety is inappropriate and can become an overwhelming, incapacitating part of a person's life.

Anxiety is slightly more common in women, adolescents, and the elderly. It can take many forms. For instance, anxiety can be characterized by sudden panic attacks, creating symptoms such as very rapid shallow breathing, sweating, palpitations, chest pains, a feeling of impending doom, or a sense of choking.

A condition known as generalized anxiety disorder is an ongoing condition characterized by bitterness, apprehension, inability to concentrate, and sleep disturbances. You may be described by your friends as constantly being on edge, impatient, and irritable. Often this type of anxiety is associated with some degree of depression and physical complaints such as headaches, muscle tension, stomachaches, palpitations, and various aches and pains.

If I do have anxiety, is there any help my doctor can give me?

There are currently a number of effective treatments for people who suffer from anxiety. The most important thing to know about the therapy, however, is that anxiety is generally a symptom, not a disease. There is something going on within you causing it and thus your physical complaints. The primary aim of therapy is to try to uncover the underlying factors.

Drug therapy has a place in the treatment of anxiety for some people. If you are physically well and your anxiety seems to have been precipitated by a definite event, such as the death of a family member, divorce, or loss of your job, then your physician may want to prescribe minor tranquilizers or anti-anxiety medications to help you cope over a short period of time. These drugs will help calm you down, but almost all of them are potentially habit forming and should be used with great caution by both your physician and you.

Most cases of anxiety can be helped with counseling or psychotherapy. Through counseling with a trained physician or specialist, you may be able to uncover the basis of the anxiety, handle the causes better, and thus control your symptoms.

There are also many things you can do to help yourself if you suffer from anxiety. If you are aware of what is causing you stress, you may be able to remove the cause. For example, if you have been in a stressful job for many years, it may be time to calmly think through the possibility of a career change. If your anxiety has been created by a stressful home life, perhaps it's time you and your spouse sought professional marriage counseling.

One of the best treatments for anxiety in almost all patients is the use of exercise. Physical exercise is a wonderful reliever of stress. You can also learn muscle-relaxation techniques to help you handle anxiety-provoking situations when they do occur.

DEPRESSION

What is depression?

Depression is a common response to events and circumstances that occur in our lives almost every day. Even though all of us will feel down or blue from time to time, depression becomes a problem when it interferes with normal social, occupational, or family life. Depression is estimated to affect over 30 million Americans.

Some of the more common symptoms of depression are an inability to concentrate, poor sleep patterns (such as being able to fall asleep, but waking up early in the morning and not being able to go back to sleep), a loss of appetite, a loss of the desire to do certain things you have always done, and crying spells.

Depression can also cause people to be physically ill. Some of the most common symptoms are physical complaints of the digestive system, frequent headaches, nervousness, and a sense of not feeling well.

Depression is the underlying cause for a great majority of symptoms reported to physicians. It is their job to make sure that there is no physical problem causing the symptoms and then, and only then, to explore the possibility that depression may be the underlying cause of the symptoms.

Is depression something I have to live with or can it be treated?

The most important part of the evaluation for depression is to recognize that it can be present. Good physicians will never assume that a patient's complaints are depression without making sure that other, more quickly curable causes are not present. For instance, a patient who comes in feeling tired or fatigued and gives many of the symptoms of depression should probably undergo a brief physical examination to determine the general level of health. Anemia, low thyroid, chronic infection, and many other physical problems can cause these same symptoms. If, in fact, no obvious cause can be found, the physician will then consider the possibility that underlying depression is playing a major role.

If hidden depression is found, it should be openly discussed with the patient. It is extremely important that the physician and the patient have an open and honest rapport. The patient may not want to hear that depression is the cause (it's more socially acceptable to be anemic), but it is important for the individual to listen and try to keep an open mind regarding suggested approaches.

Depression can be caused by obvious events, such as the death of a family member, divorce, or the sudden loss of a job. Many times through the proper counseling with a physician, a pastor, or a trained psychologist, you can learn to cope with and live with the event. Often after 2 to 3 months, the depression will clear almost as rapidly as it occurred, and you can get on with your life.

However, many people have underlying depression that stems from years and years of built-up frustrations. This type of depression should be handled by a trained specialist. It will require counseling to find some of the underlying causes and learn techniques to deal with them.

ANTIDEPRESSANTS

What are antidepressants?

Medications called antidepressants can be used to significantly relieve the symptoms. Although there are many forms of antidepressants a frequently used classification is the tricyclic. A commonly held theory is that in people with depression certain chemical imbalances occur within the brain. If these chemical imbalances are returned to normal with the use of these antidepressant medications, many of the symptoms can be relieved. Tricyclic drugs are prescribed by your physician to be taken on a regular basis for a certain period of time depending upon the amount of depression you have. The most effective approach with severely depressed patients is to combine psychotherapy with an antidepressant.

What are some of the side effects of these antidepressants?

A common side effect of antidepressant medicine is a feeling of sleepiness or grogginess in the mornings. Because most antidepressants are taken at night (they also help you sleep), the early morning hours can be a rough time for 4 to 5 days. You may experience a feeling of drunkenness, a cobwebby feeling, or drowsiness that lasts through the morning. This occurs because your system is adjusting to the drug.

If, however, you continue to take the medication as your physician prescribed, this feeling should slowly go away. Antidepressant drugs differ from tranquilizers. A tranquilizer can be given for a short period of time and sometimes on an as-needed basis. However, antidepressants must be taken on a regular basis and generally for not less than 6 to 8 weeks. Another difference between tranquilizers and antidepressants is that antidepressants don't generally produce any significant improvement in how you feel for 7 to 14 days. When you begin antidepressants, you should not expect any immediate magical change.

A dry feeling in the mouth is also a common side effect. This usually gets better but sometimes persists long enough to warrant keeping some sugarless gum or sugarless candy on hand. Work closely with your doctor during the early stages of taking these medications. There is no set dosage or type of antidepressant that is appropriate for everyone. It will take a while to find the specific dose for you. Report any potential problems to your doctor. Do not stop the medication on your own.

24.

Health Problems and Traveling

WATER

Should I drink the water wherever I travel?

Throughout most of the world, you simply cannot trust the quality of available drinking water, even though the local citizenry drink it without apparent harm. All water in less-developed areas of the world needs to be treated before drinking or using it for brushing your teeth. Major hotels in very large cities overseas may treat their own water, but if you are in doubt, even in a large hotel, draw a glass of very hot water from the tap and let it cool. The water has at least been pasteurized after passing through a water heater.

Bottled water is widely available and is always a good alternative. However, be aware that a favorite pastime in some parts of the world is for local citizens to simply refill empty bottles at a local pump. Make sure that the water has been bottled where the label indicates.

Freezing does not make water safe, so ice cubes, even those in alcoholic beverages, do not assure decontaminated water.

In deciding whether or not you should drink the water, always be overly cautious. If there is any doubt in your mind whether the water is safe and free from contamination, don't drink it. An alternative is to stick to coffee and hot tea. They should be safe as long as the water used in the preparation was brought to a full boil. Local beers, wines, and soft drinks are usually safe, also.

Can I purify my own water if I'm traveling in a remote part of the world?

Various water purification techniques can be used. You may have to take along some of the materials necessary for purification, but in many instances, it is better to do that than to suffer the consequences of drinking contaminated water.

Here are some very simple water purification methods that you can use:

- Boil the water for 1 minute. Adding a pinch of salt to the boiled water will improve its taste.
- Add 2 water purification (Halazone) tablets per quart and allow the water to stand for 30 minutes.
- Add chlorine laundry bleach (4% to 6%), 2 drops per quart if the water is clear and 4 drops per quart if the water is cloudy. Allow the water to stand for 30 minutes.
- Add 2% tincture of iodine, 3 drops per quart if the water is clear and 6 drops if it is cloudy. Allow the water to stand for 30 minutes.

It may not be the best-tasting water you've ever had, but it is as close to purification as you will get in some parts of the world.

FOOD

What is the best way to avoid eating contaminated food in a foreign country?

A great pleasure in traveling to different parts of the world is tasting the different cuisines. However, a few precautions can keep a good meal from turning into a gastrointestinal nightmare.

All meat and fish dishes should be cooked well done and eaten hot to eliminate the risk of acquiring different infectious organisms. Dishes such as steak tartare, made of raw meat, raw eggs, and spices, should not be eaten. Shopping in local open air markets (such as fish markets) and cooking your own food should be avoided.

In addition to not eating undercooked meat, the traveler should avoid cold plates, custards, pastries, or other foods prepared well in advance and left to stand. Refrigeration in most parts of the world leaves much to be desired.

Dairy products should not be consumed because of the strong likelihood of infections such as tuberculosis and brucellosis. Raw eggs should also be avoided.

An interesting note is that the meals in Chinese restaurants are usually palatable and the food safely and well cooked. This has been found to be a consistent, safe pattern throughout much of the world.

DIARRHEA

What is traveler's diarrhea?

The 3 most likely disasters to befall the 20th-century traveler are lost luggage, stolen traveler's checks, and diarrhea. This type of diarrhea is also known as Turista, Montezuma's revenge, Cairo crud, and the Delhi deli.

Many of the 8 million American travelers are turning to the more exotic delights of the world's developing nations, and about ⅓ of them will have their visit interrupted by a sudden attack of traveler's diarrhea. Traveler's diarrhea is an infectious process acquired through the ingestion of contaminated food and/or water. Especially risky foods include raw vegetables, raw meat, and raw seafood. Tap ice water, unpasteurized milk or dairy products, and unpeeled fruits are also associated with increased risk.

Traveler's diarrhea typically causes 4 to 5 loose or watery stools per day, within 24 to 48 hours after arriving at your destination. It usually continues for 3 to 4 days. About 10% of the cases last 1 week, 2% last longer than 1 month, and less than 1% will last 3 months.

What causes traveler's diarrhea?

An infectious bacterium, *E. coli,* is the primary cause of traveler's diarrhea in almost all countries where surveys have been conducted. These organisms, found in fecal material, easily contaminate raw foods and water. Once in the body, these bacteria will adhere to the small intestine where they multiply and produce a toxin (poison) that causes a marked amount of diarrhea.

Are some people more prone to traveler's diarrhea than others?

Traveler's diarrhea appears to be slightly more common in young adults than in older people. The exact reason is unclear, but it may include a lack of acquired immunity, more adventurous travel and eating styles, and poor or careless eating habits. Also, people with underlying gastrointestinal problems such as irritable bowel syndrome, colitis, ulcerative colitis, and diverticulosis seem to be a little more susceptible to traveler's diarrhea.

What measures can I take to avoid getting traveler's diarrhea?

Data indicate that probably the best way to avoid traveler's diarrhea is meticulous attention to the food and beverages you consume. However, most travelers, no matter how conscientious they are, have a great deal of difficulty sticking to these dietary restrictions.

Another common option is to take Pepto-Bismol or similar products. The active ingredient in these is bismuth subsalicylate. Taking 2

310

ounces, 4 times daily, has been shown to significantly decrease the incidence of developing traveler's diarrhea (by 60% in 1 study). However, since Pepto-Bismol's active ingredient is a salicylate, like aspirin, people who are taking aspirin for arthritis or other medical conditions can potentially cause an overdose by adding the bismuth subsalicylate.

Some people advocate taking an antidiarrhea medication throughout the trip, the most common being Lomotil. However, some controlled studies find that the active ingredient in Lomotil can actually increase the chances of developing traveler's diarrhea. The exact reason for this is unknown.

There has also been a great deal of discussion as to whether or not taking 1 of 2 different types of antibiotics can significantly reduce your chances of developing traveler's diarrhea. The antibiotic doxycycline has been shown to reduce the chances by 50% to 80%. Another medication, trimethoprim-sulfamethoxazole, also seems to be effective. However, the potential benefits must be weighed against the potential drawbacks, such as the risk of allergic reactions and the risk that some degree of intestinal upset can be caused by the antibiotic itself.

If you are a frequent traveler and are concerned about developing traveler's diarrhea, you should consult your physician about the proper preventive measures you can take.

IMMUNIZATION

Will I need any immunizations before traveling?

It will depend upon the part of the world you're going to visit and your current immunization status. The accepted rule is that developed locations—Europe, America, Japan, and England—require only a current proof of immunization for tetanus and polio.

The problem regarding immunizations comes into play when people are traveling to remote parts of the world because the diseases that are unheard of in the United States may be frequent in underdeveloped areas. We rarely hear of malaria in the United States, but it is a significant problem in certain parts of Asia; therefore, people traveling there should make sure they are protected against developing malaria.

It would be impossible for me to give the exact recommendations for each part of the world, so you should contact your local physician, local public health department (ask for United States government pamphlet *Health Information for International Travel*), or the Centers for Disease Control, the Division of Quarantine, in Atlanta, Georgia, to get specific information regarding the immunizations you will need. A word of caution: Contact them at least 2 to 3 months prior to your trip to make sure you have adequate time to get the shots you might need.

ALTITUDE SICKNESS

Why do I get sick every time I go up in the mountains?

Sports such as skiing, hiking, trekking, and climbing have become so popular that several hundred thousand people each year transfer themselves from their normal low-altitude homes to the high elevations of the mountains. Because many do not understand the effects that elevation can have on their health, thousands develop illnesses related to the altitude.

The effects that altitude can have upon health have to do with the oxygen content in the air. At lower elevations, nearer sea level, there is enough oxygen in the air to meet all bodily needs. However, as we ascend into higher elevations, the air becomes "thinner" and contains less oxygen. At some critical point (around 8000'), there is simply not enough oxygen in the air to adequately supply our needs. If, when we reach this altitude, we are not aware of the potential problem and do not take precautions, we can develop a variety of symptoms—collectively known as altitude sickness.

The extent of the possible altitude sickness depends upon 4 factors: (1) the speed at which the altitude is achieved; (2) the altitude reached; (3) the duration of the stay; and (4) individual characteristics. The effects of high altitude can be anything from unexplained fatigue to severe headache to an acute life-threatening problem in which the lungs fill up with fluid. Understanding the basic reasons for this and knowing how to prevent it are critical to anyone traveling to higher altitudes.

What is the most common form of altitude sickness?

Acute mountain sickness is the most common form of altitude sickness. It is quite unpleasant and usually causes you to miss 24 to 48 hours of your particular activity.

The most frequent symptoms are headache, weakness, nausea, shortness of breath, and disturbed sleep that tend to get worse when combined with fatigue, jet lag, excessive amounts of alcohol, or underlying medical problems. Common-sense medicine—rest and relieving the symptoms—will allow the problem to subside.

High-altitude pulmonary edema is a much more serious form of acute altitude sickness, generally occurring in young children, young adults, and older people. People can develop acute shortness of breath, fol-

312

lowed by an accumulation of fluid within the lungs that, left untreated, can lead to serious consequences.

High-altitude pulmonary edema, although much less common than other forms, begins as a severe headache and can rapidly lead to mental confusion, hallucinations, difficulty in walking, and death.

What are some of the ways that I can keep from having altitude sickness?

A good way to lessen your chances of developing altitude sickness is simply to understand that it can occur. Any time you are traveling to higher elevations, you need to be aware of preventive measures.

Do not overeat, drink too much, or become fatigued during your trip to the mountains. Upon arrival at your destination, especially if it is over 8000′, take things slow—rest for the 1st 24 hours and don't overdo. Avoid alcoholic beverages for the 1st 48 hours, and after that, consume them only in moderation. If you are a cigarette smoker, you should seriously consider stopping or severely curtailing the number of cigarettes you smoke during your visit.

Only after a period of allowing your body to acclimatize to the new altitude should you begin any strenuous activity such as skiing. For those who are going to do any climbing in the higher elevations: take the climb slowly. Allow 4 days to climb 10,000′ and 1 day for each additional 1000′ above that. Trying to push yourself too fast and too far at higher elevations can lead to serious consequences.

MOTION SICKNESS

Is there any way I can prevent motion sickness?

Motion sickness, often a severe problem for people traveling by air, sea, and even land, results because of an imbalance created in the inner ear. This imbalance can cause severe dizziness, vertigo, nausea, and vomiting.

The most practical method for reducing your chances of developing motion sickness is the use of proper medications. Antimotion sickness tablets can be taken 3 to 4 days before you leave and continued throughout your trip. Medications such as Antivert and Dramamine have been used with varying degrees of success by many people.

A newer method for the prevention of motion sickness is a small patch containing the chemical scopolamine (an effective antimotion sickness medication) that is placed behind the ear. A scopolamine patch can deliver enough medication throughout the day to prevent motion

313

sickness. Placed behind the ear prior to traveling, the patch will last for approximately 3 days. It keeps a constant level of medication in the system.

There are, however, some other helpful hints that could significantly reduce your chances of developing motion sickness:
• Take medications as prescribed by your physician.
• Have a fairly fixed visual point, such as the horizon.
• Avoid staring at 1 place too long.
• At sea, always stay amidships.
• Do not overindulge in food or drink, and do not smoke.
• Stay in well-ventilated areas.
• Avoid stress, fatigue, and unpleasant surroundings as much as possible.

FLYING

Should certain people avoid air travel?

The potential medical consequences of air travel make it mandatory that certain people be advised not to fly. Among them are those who have suffered an acute heart attack within the previous 4 weeks or a stroke in the previous 2 weeks, people with uncontrolled hypertension, anyone who has had surgical wiring of the jaw (because of the possibility of vomiting due to motion sickness), poorly controlled epileptics, severe anemics (especially with sickle-cell anemia), and anyone who is more than 240 days pregnant. Also in this category is the severe chronic lung patient who requires oxygen at all times. Although special arrangements can be made for these people, they should select other means of travel if at all possible.

Why do my ears hurt when I travel by plane?

Although the cabins on jet airplanes are pressurized, the systems cannot maintain pressure equal to that at ground level. These aircraft fly between 28,000' and 45,000' but they can maintain cabin pressure equivalent to only 5000' to 8000' feet altitude. When you are flying in a jet, you are sitting in an atmosphere similar to that found on an 8000' mountain.

Because of this, pressure created within the cabin can affect your ears and sinuses. Normally, pressure behind the eardrum in the middle ear is maintained at a constant level because of a small tube (the eustachian tube) connecting it and the back of the throat. If the eustachian tube is functioning properly, the pressure within the airplane will equal that within the middle ear, and there is no pressure buildup. However, if you have had a bad cold, congestion, or allergies, the eustachian tube can close up and make the inner ear pressure and the airplane cabin pressure unequal. The negative, or lower, pressure behind the eardrum can cause a sensation of fullness, pressure, and intense pain. If this condition becomes severe, a condition known as barotitis media can occur and can cause rupture of the eardrum and deafness.

How can I avoid developing this problem with my ears?

In the Air Force, the standard rule is: "never fly when you have a cold." In high-performance aircraft, flying with a cold may not only be very painful, but it can interfere with the pilot's ability to command the aircraft. This is a bit extreme for civilian travelers, but I can certainly caution you about flying when you have a cold.

Anyone who has suffered a recent cold, especially someone with a feeling of pressure, popping, or clicking in the ears, should begin taking some form of decongestant/antihistamine preparation 3 to 4 days prior to flying. This gives the medication a chance to open up the eustachian tube before you get on the plane.

In flight, many adults can achieve a temporary opening of the eustachian tube by swallowing, coughing, chewing gum, and moving the lower jaw from side to side.

Children are especially prone to this problem. If your child develops a feeling of fullness or pain in the ear while flying, encourage the child to drink from a bottle, suck on a pacifier, chew gum (if old enough), or continually drink fluids.

If none of these tricks works then equalize the pressure by using Valsalva's maneuver. Hold the nose and mouth shut and forcefully puff out the cheeks. The purpose is to trap air and force it back up the eustachian tube.

People who experience recurrent episodes of pressure related problems during air travel should consult their physician for a more intensive regimen of medication before flying.

TRAVEL AND YOUR CHILD

Is there any advice you can offer about how to travel with children?

When you are traveling with children, it is definitely the little things that count. There are some general tips that can make traveling with your children more enjoyable for everyone.

Never travel with a sick child. Many parents will feel that even though the child is sick, they are still going to go on their vacation. This is unfair to the child and to the family, because sick children simply do not travel well.

Spend some time prior to the trip organizing the time your child will spend traveling. Make sure your child has some toys, crayons and coloring books and, with older children, an adequate supply of good reading material. You can also plan to play games with your child, such as counting cows or naming the ABC's using billboards. All of these involve your child in the trip and avoid the hassles that come when the child is bored.

When you eat in restaurants, avoid the rush hours—children do best when they eat slowly and methodically. Rush-hour traffic in a restaurant can provide the children with an excellent opportunity to get into trouble and the parents an excellent chance to develop an ulcer.

A common problem with children, especially on long car trips, is motion sickness. For older children (above 3 years of age), medications such as Benadryl and Dramamine can be used in dosages recommended by your physician. In addition, there are a few simple preventive measures that can lessen the chance of developing motion sickness in any traveler:

- You can try traveling at night when visual stimulation is reduced, or have your children wear dark sunglasses for daytime travel.
- *Unless your child is a seasoned traveler,* don't let him or her read in a moving vehicle. This can cause eyestrain and headaches as well as motion sickness.
- Make sure there is adequate ventilation in the car while traveling. Rolling down a window just a few inches can provide enough fresh air to reduce the chance of motion sickness.
- If your child is susceptible to motion sickness, the best place to ride is strapped into a child safety seat or seat belt in the middle of the backseat.

Traveling with children should add to a vacation, not take away from it. However, it is the parents' responsibility to plan to travel with children rather than simply throw them in the backseat of the car and expect everything to go okay.

EMERGENCY MEDICAL KIT

What are some of the things that I should put in a medicine kit in case of an emergency?

Vacation should be a time to get away from all of our troubles. Yet, many people spend days planning the hotel they will stay in but not a moment on how to prevent or be prepared for potential health problems. With a little bit of planning, medical concerns can be kept to a minimum.

If you are going to an out-of-the-way place where medical care will be hard to find, take along a medical kit. Of course, you can't anticipate everything, but there are some generally accepted things that you should include in this kit.

Make sure that you have a nonallergic soap, antiseptic cream, and bandages for cuts and scrapes.

If you are traveling with children, have some aspirin or acetaminophen for unexpected fevers.

Since traveling seems to upset many people's stomachs and digestive systems, it is a good idea to have some medications for diarrhea and constipation.

Take a sunscreen to protect you and your children from sunburn.

If you are going to the mountains, a ready-made splint is a must.

If you are on any medications prescribed by your physician, have enough to last the duration of the trip plus 1 extra week in case your trip is unexpectedly prolonged.

HEART DISEASE

Should people with heart disease take any precautions when traveling?

People with cardiovascular disease such as angina or hypertension and people who have had a stroke can travel, but there are some special considerations that should be noted.

Remember that travel needs to be postponed for at least 2 weeks following recovery from a stroke and a minimum of 4 weeks following a heart attack.

In scheduling trips, people with these conditions will want to allow ample time for getting from place to place and avoid rushing, stress, and fatigue.

People with heart disease who travel by air, especially those with a history of blood clots in the legs, should wear elastic support hose in flight and avoid prolonged periods of sitting. Getting up frequently and strolling down the aisle will help prevent cramping in the legs.

Anyone who has suffered from attacks of severe shortness of breath will need to make arrangements with the airline at least 3 to 4 days prior to flight time to ensure the availability of an extra supply of oxygen on board.

Because the low humidity of the pressurized cabin can contribute to mild dehydration, people with heart disease should drink extra fluids during the trip. But avoid alcoholic beverages.

When traveling across more than 1 time zone, the effects of jet lag can set in. This can be especially taxing to the person with heart disease; the individual should rest for at least 1 to 2 days upon arrival before beginning any social or travel commitments.

A word of caution for anyone with heart disease. If you are on medication, make sure that you have an adequate supply before you leave. I strongly recommend that you take the medication needed for the trip *plus* enough for 1 extra week. If you are traveling abroad, it's best to take at least an extra month's supply just in case travel arrangements are delayed. In many places, it is extremely difficult to get prescriptions filled.

JET LAG

Is jet lag a real problem, or is it just a myth?

Over the past several years, I have had the opportunity to travel throughout the country, and I can tell you that jet lag is a fact, not a myth. Jet lag is actually caused by changes that occur in our normal body rhythms when we travel across multiple time zones.

We all have an internal biological clock that governs how we feel, the times we sleep, and how our bodies react to the pressures of everyday life. When we travel across time zones, the internal clock malfunctions and is not able to adjust immediately to the new changes.

Jet lag is generally characterized by fatigue, alterations of normal eating patterns, changes in kidney and bowel functions, sleep disturbances, and marked difficulty in mental and physical performance.

Adjustments in the body's internal clock, the circadian rhythm, generally takes 24 to 48 hours. The length of time that it takes to adjust to jet lag tends to increase when the travel is in an eastward rather than a westward direction. The explanation for this may lie in the fact that eastward travel results in a shorter day and most circadian rhythms have cycles of approximately 24 hours. As we travel westward, the day is actually lengthened, and the adjustment is a little easier.

Jet lag is a problem to even seasoned travelers when they are expected to perform at their peak immediately after arriving at their new destination.

Any suggestions on how I can best handle jet lag?

The symptoms of jet lag can be minimized if the traveler takes a few precautionary steps—prior to and during the trip:

- Readjust your sleep patterns before you begin your trip. If you are traveling from east to west, you should go to bed a little later every night and arise later, starting about 3 days before your trip.
- When traveling from west to east, you should go to sleep earlier and get up earlier for 3 days prior to your trip.
- Make sure that you get a good night's rest the night before you leave.
- If you are traveling over more than 4 or 5 time zones, schedule stop-overs instead of nonstop flights if you can.
- While traveling in the airplane, exercise in your seat and stand or move about the cabin whenever possible. Deep breathing, moving your legs, raising your knees, turning your head, swinging your arms overhead, and relaxing and contracting the muscles in the lower legs can improve your adjustment.
- Adjust you meal schedule gradually before departing. Begin about a week before leaving on a long trip so that by the time you leave you are actually eating on the time schedule of your destination.
- Try to avoid tension and stress during the flight.
- Don't overeat during the flight. Keep alcohol to a minimum.

After you arrive at your destination, don't cut yourself short on sleep. Many people will try to immediately adjust to the new time zone and lose effective sleep. Take 24 to 48 hours to adjust to the new time zone before beginning a vigorous vacation. Make sure that you keep plenty of fluids in your system because the humidity of the airplane has actually caused some degree of dehydration and that fluid must be replaced.

Index

322